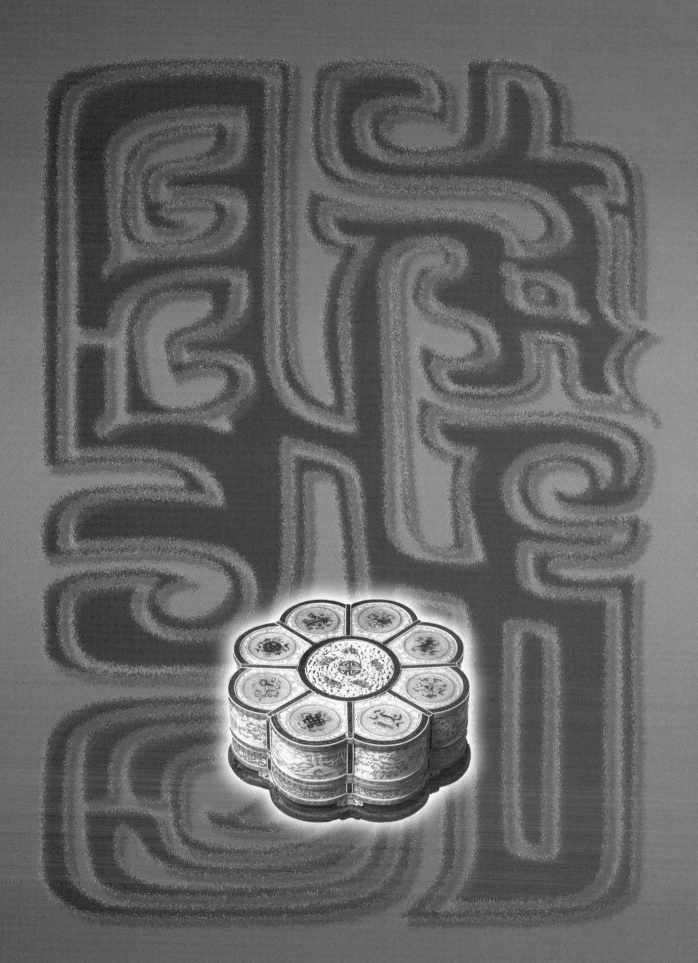

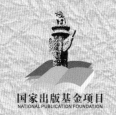

国家出版基金项目
NATIONAL PUBLICATION FOUNDATION

中华医药卫生

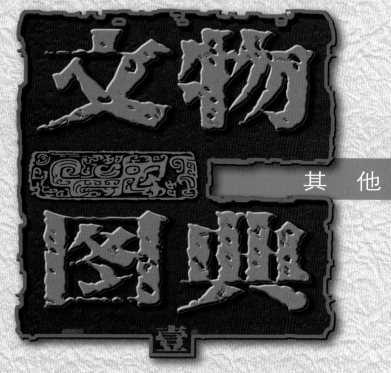

其 他 卷

主 编　李经纬　梁　峻　刘学春
总主译　白永权
主 译　杜彦龙

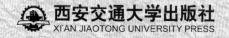

西安交通大学出版社
XI'AN JIAOTONG UNIVERSITY PRESS

图书在版编目（CIP）数据

中华医药卫生文物图典 . 1. 其他卷 . / 李经纬，梁峻，
刘学春主编 .— 西安：西安交通大学出版社，2016.12

ISBN 978-7-5605-7020-4

Ⅰ . ①中… Ⅱ . ①李… ②梁… ③刘… Ⅲ . ①中国医药学—
文物—中国—图录 Ⅳ . ① R-092 ② K870.2

中国版本图书馆 CIP 数据核字（2015）第 022430 号

书　　名	中华医药卫生文物图典（一）其他卷
主　　编	李经纬　梁　峻　刘学春
责任编辑	郭泉泉

出版发行	西安交通大学出版社
	（西安市兴庆南路 10 号　邮政编码 710049）
网　　址	http://www.xjtupress.com
电　　话	（029）82668805　82668502（医学分社）
	（029）82668315（总编办）
传　　真	（029）82668280
印　　刷	中煤地西安地图制印有限公司

开　　本	889mm×1194mm　1/16　印张 31.5　字数 524 千字
版次印次	2017 年 12 月第 1 版　2017 年 12 月第 1 次印刷
书　　号	ISBN 978-7-5605-7020-4
定　　价	980.00 元

读者购书、书店添货、如发现印装质量问题，请通过以下方式联系、调换。

订购热线：（029）82665248　（029）82665249

投稿热线：（029）82668805　（029）82668502

读者信箱：medpress@126.com

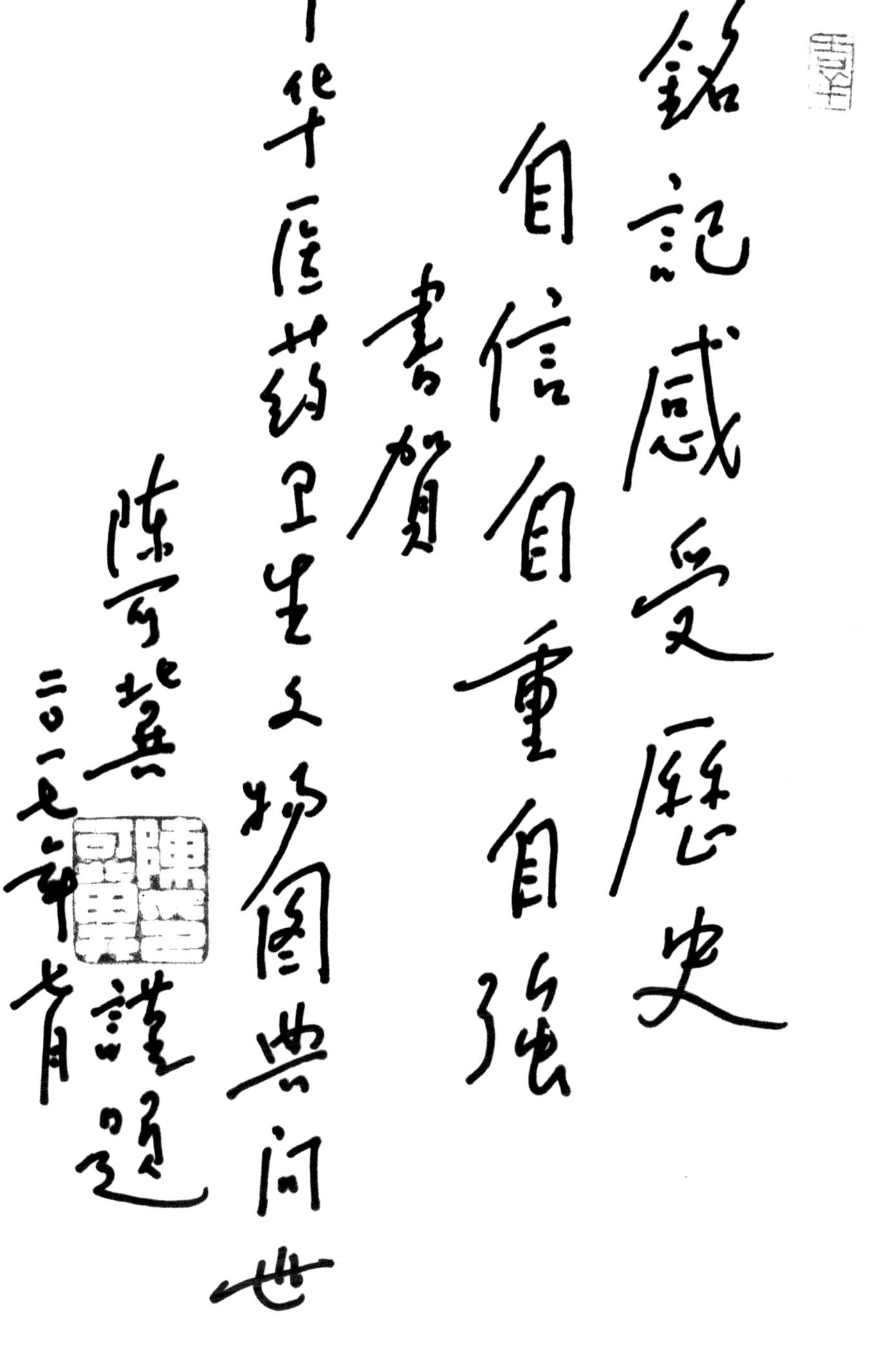

铭记感受历史

自信自重自强

书贺

中华医药卫生文物图典问世

陈可冀 谨题

二〇二七年肖

陈可冀　中国科学院院士、国医大师

精修醫藥衛生文物

圖典功著當代

深究岐黃學術思想

淵源惠澤千秋

中華醫藥衛生文物圖典出版誌慶

丁酉孟秋 孫光榮 敬題於北京

孫光荣　国医大师

中華醫藥衛生文物圖典出版

彰顯中醫藥
文化精神

體現中醫藥
歷史價值

歲次丁酉夏 王琦

王琦　国医大师

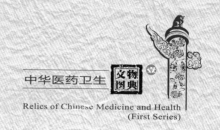

中华医药卫生文物图典（一）
丛书编撰委员会

主　编　李经纬　梁　峻　刘学春

副主编　廖　果　吴鸿洲　康兴军　和中浚　刘小斌　杨金生

　　　　郑怀林　徐江雁　白建疆　黄　煌

编　委　李洪晓　梁永宣　王强虎　董树平　马　健　王　霞

　　　　张雅宗　朱德明　包哈申　张建青　郑　蓉　庄乾竹

　　　　李宏红　刘哲峰　王宏才　陈润东

总主译　白永权

主　译　陈向京　聂文信　范晓晖　温　睿　赵永生　杜彦龙

　　　　吉　乐　李小棉　郭　梦　陈　曦

副主译（按姓氏音序排列）

　　　　董艳云　姜雨孜　李建西　刘　慧　马　健　任宝磊

　　　　任　萌　任　莹　王　颇　习通源　谢皖吉　徐素云

　　　　许崇钰　许　梅　詹菊红　赵　菲　邹郝晶

译　者（按姓氏音序排列）

迟征宇　邓　甜　付一豪　高　琛　高　媛　郭　宁

韩　蕾　何宗昌　胡勇强　黄　鋆　蒋新蕾　康晓薇

李静波　刘雅恬　刘妍萌　鲁显生　马　月　牛笑语

唐云鹏　唐臻娜　田　多　铁红玲　佟健一　王　晨

王　丹　王　栋　王　丽　王　媛　王慧敏　王梦杰

王仙先　吴耀均　席　慧　肖国强　许子洋　闫红贤

杨姣姣　姚　晔　张　阳　张　鋆　张继飞　张梦原

张晓谦　赵　欣　赵亚力　郑　青　郑艳华　朱江嵩

朱瑛培

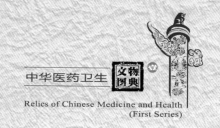

中华医药卫生 文物图典

Relics of Chinese Medicine and Health
(First Series)

本册编撰委员会

主　编	李经纬　梁　峻　刘学春
副主编	廖　果　吴鸿洲　康兴军　和中浚　刘小斌　杨金生
	郑怀林　徐江雁　白建疆　黄　煌
编　委	李洪晓　梁永宣　王强虎　董树平　马　健　王　霞
	张雅宗　朱德明　包哈申　张建青　郑　蓉　庄乾竹
	李宏红　刘哲峰　王宏才　陈润东

总主译	白永权
主　译	杜彦龙
副主译	刘　慧
译　者	谢皖吉　康晓薇

丛书策划委员会

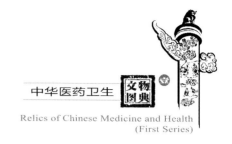

中华医药卫生 文物图典

Relics of Chinese Medicine and Health
(First Series)

序 言

　　探索天、地、人运动变化规律以及"气化物生"过程的相互关系，是人类永恒的课题。宇宙不可逆，地球不可逆，人生不可逆业已成为共识。天地造化形成自然，人类活动构成文化。文物既是文化的载体，又是物化的历史，还是文明的见证。

　　追求健康长寿是人类共同的夙愿。中华民族之所以繁衍昌盛，健康文化起了巨大的推动作用。由于古人谋求生存发展、应对环境变化产生的智慧，大多反映在以医药卫生为核心的健康文化之中，所以，习总书记说："中医药学是中国古代科学的瑰宝，也是打开中华文明宝库的钥匙"。

　　秉持文化大发展、大繁荣理念，中国中医科学院李经纬、梁峻等为负责人的科研团队在完成科技部"国家重点医药卫生文物收集调研和保护"课题获 2005 年度中华中医药学会科技二等奖基础上，又资鉴"夏商周断代工程""中华文明探源工程"等相关考古成果，用有重要价值的新出土文物置换原拍摄质量较差的文物，适当补充民族医药文物，共精选收载 5000 余件。经西安交通大学出版社申报，《中华医药卫生文物图典（一）》（以下简称《图典》）于 2013 年获得了国家出版基金的资助，并经专业翻译团队翻译，使《图典》得以面世。

　　文物承载的信息多元丰富，发掘解读其中蕴藏的智慧并非易事。医药卫生文物更具有特殊性，除文物的一般属性外，还承载着传统医学发展史迹与促进健康的信息。运用历史唯物主义观察发掘文物信息，善于从生活文物中领悟卫生信息，才能准确解读其功能，也才能诠释其在民生健康中的历史作用，收到以古鉴今之效果。"历史是现实的根源"，任何一个民族都不能割断历史，史料都包含在文化中。"文化是民族的血脉，是人民的精神家园"，文化繁荣才能实现中华民族的伟大复兴。值本《图典》付梓之际，用"梳理文化之脉，必获健康之果"作为序言并和作者、读者共勉！

中央文史研究馆馆员
中国工程院院士　　王永炎
丁酉年仲夏

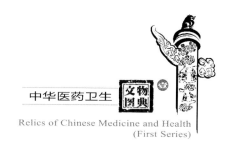

中华医药卫生 文物图典

Relics of Chinese Medicine and Health
(First Series)

序　言

　　探索天、地、人运动变化规律以及"气化物生"过程的相互关系，是人类永恒的课题。宇宙不可逆，地球不可逆，人生不可逆业已成为共识。天地造化形成自然，人类活动构成文化。文物既是文化的载体，又是物化的历史，还是文明的见证。

　　追求健康长寿是人类共同的夙愿。中华民族之所以繁衍昌盛，健康文化起了巨大的推动作用。由于古人谋求生存发展、应对环境变化产生的智慧，大多反映在以医药卫生为核心的健康文化之中，所以，习总书记说："中医药学是中国古代科学的瑰宝，也是打开中华文明宝库的钥匙"。

　　秉持文化大发展、大繁荣理念，中国中医科学院李经纬、梁峻等为负责人的科研团队在完成科技部"国家重点医药卫生文物收集调研和保护"课题获 2005 年度中华中医药学会科技二等奖基础上，又资鉴"夏商周断代工程""中华文明探源工程"等相关考古成果，用有重要价值的新出土文物置换原拍摄质量较差的文物，适当补充民族医药文物，共精选收载 5000 余件。经西安交通大学出版社申报，《中华医药卫生文物图典（一）》（以下简称《图典》）于 2013 年获得了国家出版基金的资助，并经专业翻译团队翻译，使《图典》得以面世。

　　文物承载的信息多元丰富，发掘解读其中蕴藏的智慧并非易事。 医药卫生文物更具有特殊性，除文物的一般属性外，还承载着传统医学发展史迹与促进健康的信息。运用历史唯物主义观察发掘文物信息，善于从生活文物中领悟卫生信息，才能准确解读其功能，也才能诠释其在民生健康中的历史作用，收到以古鉴今之效果。"历史是现实的根源"，任何一个民族都不能割断历史，史料都包含在文化中。"文化是民族的血脉，是人民的精神家园"，文化繁荣才能实现中华民族的伟大复兴。值本《图典》付梓之际，用"梳理文化之脉，必获健康之果"作为序言并和作者、读者共勉！

中央文史研究馆馆员
中国工程院院士　　王永炎
丁酉年仲夏

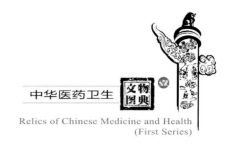

中华医药卫生 文物图典

Relics of Chinese Medicine and Health
(First Series)

前 言

文化是相对自然的概念，是考古界常用词汇。文物是文化的重要组成部分，既是文明的物证，又是物化的历史。狭义医药卫生文物是疾病防治模式语境下的解读，而广义医药卫生文物则是躯体、心态、环境适应三维健康模式下的诠释。中华民族是56个民族组成的多元一体大家庭，中华医药卫生文物当然包括各民族的健康文化遗存。

天地造化如造山、板块漂移、气候变迁、生物起源进化等形成自然。气化物生莫贵于人，即整个生物进化的最高成果是人类自身。广义而言，人类生存思维留下的痕迹即物质财富和精神财富总和构成文化，其一般的物化形式是视觉感知的文物、文献、胜迹等。其中质变标志明晰的文化如文字、文物、城市、礼仪等可称作文明。从唯物史观视角观察，狭义文化即精神财富，尤其体现人类精、气、神状态的事项，其本质也具有特殊物质属性，如量子也具有波粒二相性，这种粒子也是物质，无非运动方式特殊而已。现代所谓可重复验证的"科学"，事实上也是从文化中分离出来的事项，因此也是一种特殊文化形式。追求健康长寿是人类共同的夙愿。中华民族之所以繁衍昌盛，是因为健康文化异彩纷呈。中华优秀传统医药文化之所以博大精深，是因为其原创思维博大、格物致知精深，所以，习总书记说："中医药学是中国古代科学的瑰宝，也是打开中华文明宝库的钥匙"。

文化既反映时代、地域、民族分布、生产资料来源、技术水平等信息，又反映人类认知水平和生存智慧。发掘解读文物、文献中蕴藏的健康知识和灵动智慧，首先是从事健康工作者的责任和义务。《易经》设有"观"卦，人类作为观察者，不仅要积极收藏展陈文物，而且要善于捕捉文物倾诉的信息，汲取养分，启迪思维，收到古为今用之效果。墨子三表法，首先一表即"本之于古者圣王之事"，也是强调古代史实的重要性。"历史是现实的根源"，现实是未来的基础。任何一个国家、地区、民族都不能割断历史、忽略基础，这个基础就是文化。"文化是民族的血脉，是人民的精神家园"。文化繁荣才能驱动各项事业发展，才能实现中华民族的伟大复兴。

人类从类人猿分化出来。"禄丰古猿禄丰种"是云南禄丰发现的类人猿化石，距今七八百万年。距今200万年前人类进入旧石器时代，直立行走，打制石器产生工具意识，管理火种，是所谓"燧人氏"时代。中国留存有更新世早、中期的元谋、蓝田、北京人等遗址。距今10万—5万年前，人类进入旧石器时代中期，即早期智人阶段，脑容量增加，和欧洲、非洲人种相比，原始蒙古人种颧骨前突等，是所谓"伏羲氏"时代。中国发现的马坝、长阳、丁村人等较典型。距今5万—1万年前，人类进入旧石器时代晚期，即晚期智人阶段，细石器、骨角器等遍布全国，山顶洞、柳江、资阳人等较典型。

中石器时代距今约1万年，是旧石器时代向新石器时代的短暂过渡期，弓箭发明，狗被驯化。河南灵井、陕西沙苑遗址等作为代表。距今1万—公元前2600年前后，人类进入新石器时代，磨光石器、烧制陶器，出现农业村落并饲养家畜，是所谓"神农氏"时代。公元前7000年以来，在甲、骨、陶、石等载体上出现契刻符号、七音阶骨笛乐器等，反映出人文气息趋浓。公元前6000—公元前3500年的老官台、裴李岗、河姆渡、马家浜、仰韶等文化遗址，彰显出先民围绕生存健康问题所做的各种努力。

公元前4800年以来，以关中、晋南、豫西为中心形成的仰韶文化，是中原史前文化的重要标志。以半坡、庙底沟类型为典型，自公元前3500年走向繁荣，属于锄耕粟黍稻兼营渔猎饲养猪鸡经济方式，彩陶尤其发达。公元前4400—公元前3300年，长江中游的大溪文化，薄胎彩陶和白陶发达。公元前4300—公元前2500年山东丰岛的大汶口文化，红陶为主。公元前3500年前后，辽东的红山文化原始宗教发展。公元前 3300 年以来，长江下游由河姆渡、马家浜文化衍续的良渚文化和陇西的马家窑文化、江淮间的薛家岗文化时趋发达。

公元前 2600—公元前 2000 年，黄河中下游龙山文化群形成，冶铸铜器，制作玉器，土坯、石灰、夯筑技术开始应用。公元前 2697 年，轩辕战败炎帝（有说其后裔）、蚩尤而为黄帝纪元元年。黄帝西巡访贤，"至岐见岐伯，引载而归，访于治道"。其引归地"溱洧襟带于前，梅泰环拱于后"，即今河南新密市古城寨。岐黄答问，构建《黄帝内经》健康知识体系，中华文明从关注民生健康起步。颛顼改革宗教，神职人员出现；帝喾修身节用，帝尧和合百国，舜同律度量衡，大禹疏导治水，中华民族不断繁衍昌盛。

公元前 2070 年，禹之子启以豫西晋南为中心建立夏王朝，二里头青铜文化为其特征，半地穴、窑洞、地面建筑并存。饮食卫生器具、酒器增多。朱砂安神作用在宫殿应用。公元前 1600 年，商灭夏。偃师商城设有铸铜作坊。公元前 1300 年，盘庚迁殷，使用甲骨文。武丁时期青铜浑铸、分铸并存。公元前 1056 年，相传周"文王被殷纣拘于姜里，演《周易》，成六十四卦"。公元前 1046 年，武王克商建周，定都镐京。青铜器始铸长篇铭文，周原发掘出微型甲骨文字。公元前 770 年，平王东迁。虢国铸铜柄铁剑。公元前 753 年，秦国设置史官。公元前 707 年出现蝗灾、公元前 613 年出现"哈雷彗星"，均被孔子载入《春秋》。公元前 221 年，秦始皇统一中国，多元一体民族大家庭形成，中华医药卫生文物异彩纷呈。

中国是治史大国，历来重视发展文化博物事业，1955 年成立卫生部中医研究院时就设置医史研究室，1982 年中国医史文献研究所成立时复建中国医史博物馆研究收藏展陈文物。2000—2003 年，经王永炎院士、姚乃礼院长等呼吁，科技部批准立项，由李经纬、梁峻为负责人的团队完成"国家重点医药卫生文物收集调研和保护"项目任务，受到科技部项目验收组专家的高度评价，获中华中医药学会科技进步二等奖。2013 年，在国家出版基金资助下，课题组对部分文物重新拍摄或必要置换、充实民族医药文物后，由西安交通大学出版社编辑、组聘国内一流翻译团队英译说明文字付梓，受到国家中医药博物馆筹备工作领导小组和办公室的高度重视。

"物以类聚"，《图典》主要依据文物质地、种类分为 9 卷，计有陶瓷，金属，纸质，竹木，玉石、织品及标本，壁画石刻及遗址，少数民族文物，其他，备考等卷。同卷下主要根据历史年代或小类分册设章。每卷下的历史时段不求统一。遵循上述规则将《图典》划分为21册，总计收载文物5000余件。对每件文物的描述，除质地、规格、馆藏等基本要素外，重点描述其在民生健康中的作用。对少数暂不明确的事项在括号中注明待考。对引自各博物馆的材料除在文物后列出馆藏外，还在书后再次统一列出馆名或参考书目，以充分尊重其馆藏权，也同时维护本典作者的引用权。

21世纪，围绕人类健康的生命科学将飞速发展，但科学离不开文化，文化离不开文物。发掘文物承载的信息为现实服务，谨引用横渠先生四言之两语："为天地立心，为生民立命"，既作为编撰本《图典》之宗旨，也是我们践行国家"一带一路"倡议的具体努力。希冀通过本《图典》的出版发行，教育国人，提振中华民族精神；走向世界，为人类健康事业贡献力量。

李经纬　梁峻　刘学春

2017年6月于北京

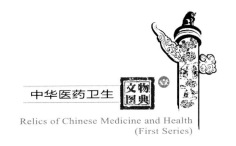

中华医药卫生 文物图典

Relics of Chinese Medicine and Health
(First Series)

目 录

第八章 清(1840年以前)

第九章　近现代

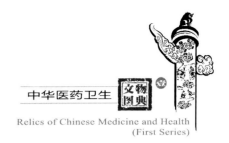

中华医药卫生 文物图典

Relics of Chinese Medicine and Health
(First Series)

Contents

Chapter Eight   Qing Dynasty

Chapter Nine   Modern Times

◈ 第一章 远古时期

Chapter One　Primitive Ages

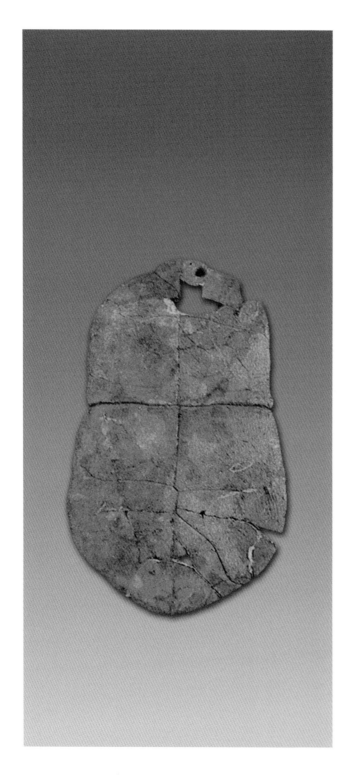

刻符龟甲

新石器时代，距今 7000 多年

骨质

长 16 厘米，宽 8.5 ~ 10 厘米

Tortoise Shell Carved with Symbols

The Neolithic Age (7000 years ago)

Bone

Length 16 cm/ Width 8.5-10 cm

上刻一个 ⬭ 形符号，与殷墟卜辞中的
"目"字较为相似，是世界上目前最早与文
字起源有关的实物资料——甲骨契刻符号，
可能具有原始文字的性质。1987年河南舞
阳贾湖出土。

河南博物院藏

The tortoise shell is inscribed with a symbol, ⬭,
resembling "目" (eye) in the oracle inscriptions of
the Yin Dynasty Ruins, which is called Jiagu
symbols, the earliest objects relating to the origin
of Chinese characters so far, so the inscription
is of the feature of primal characters. It was
unearthed in Jiahu, Wuyang County, Henan
Province, in 1987.

Preserved in Henan Museum

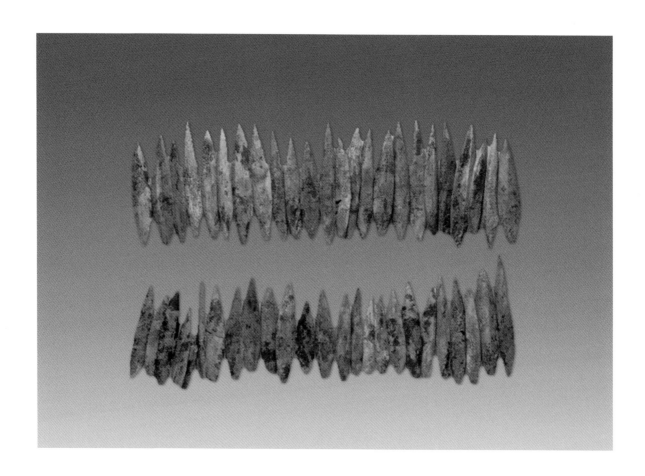

骨镞

新石器时代

骨质

平均长 6.5 厘米

Bone Arrowheads

The Neolithic Age

Bone

Average Length 6.5 cm

利用动物长骨磨制，共 49 枚，做工精细程度

不一。成排出土于 M28 椁室北端，紧贴内壁。

中国海盐博物馆藏

The arrowheads are made of the animal's long
bones through grinding and sharpening. There
are 49 in total. Some look fine and the other
look coarse. They were found in rows against
the inner wall at the northern end of the coffin
pit in Tomb M28 when unearthed.

Preserved in China Sea-salt Museum

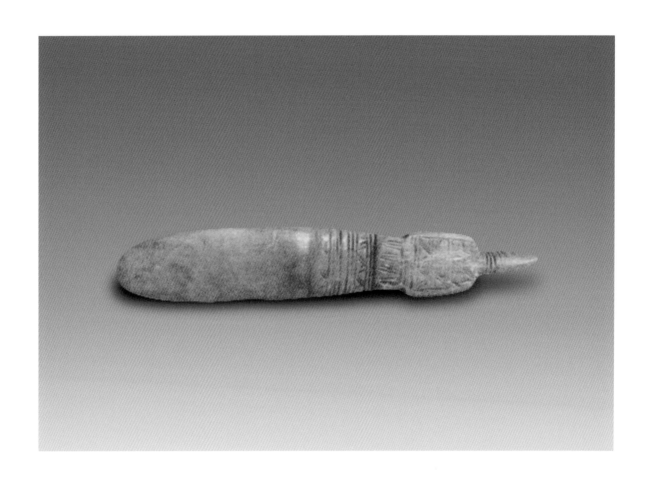

象牙雕鸟形匕

新石器时代，河姆渡文化

象牙质

长 17 厘米

Bird-shaped Ivory Carving Spoon

Hemudu Culture, the Neolithic Age

Ivory

Length 17 cm

这件匕整体雕成一只凤鸟状，圆形的柄部细而向下弯曲，柄根部有几周阳线刻出的弦纹，柄似凤鸟尖喙；匕身中部宽厚而隆起，正面刻画出弦纹与斜线纹，匕身首部渐宽而薄，端头为圆弧形上翘。雕刻技艺精美，堪称这类作品中的杰作。中国古代进食工具。1978 年浙江省余姚市河姆渡遗址出土。

浙江省博物馆藏

The spoon is carved into the shape of a phoenix with a round handle whose end becomes tapered and decurved. There are several protruding lines inscribed around the handle root. The handle is in the shape of the sharp beak of a phoenix. The middle part of the spoon is broad, thick and bulging. The obverse side is engraved with some string patterns and oblique lines. The front part becomes wide and thin gradually, with its upwarping tip in circular arc shape. The spoon, served as tableware in ancient China, is exquisitely and elegantly carved and can be rated as a masterpiece among its congener ware. It was unearthed in Hemudu Sites, Yuyao City, Zhejiang Province, in 1978.

Preserved in Zhejiang Provincial Museum

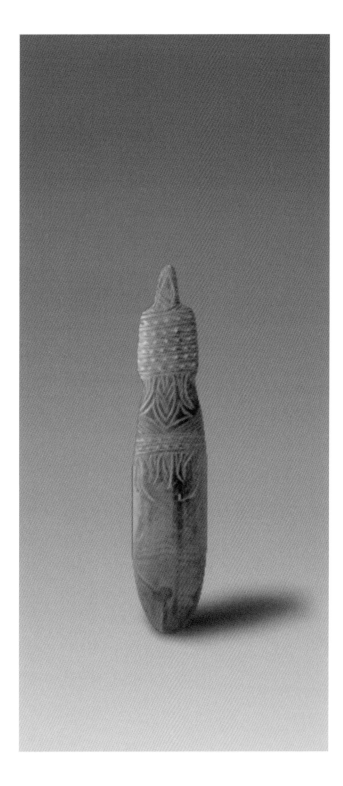

象牙鸟形匕

新石器时代，河姆渡文化

象牙质

长 13.6 厘米

Bird-shaped Ivory Spoon

Hemudu Culture, the Neolithic Age

Ivory

Length 13.6 cm

圆雕，正面呈匕形，剔刻植物纹，也可能是表现"社"的图案；侧面为飞翔的鸟的侧影；背面镂挖可供系挂的小孔。雕刻精美，制作讲究，当非一般的日用器。1996 年浙江省余姚市鲻山遗址出土。

浙江省文物考古研究所藏

The spoon is carved in the round. The obverse side is shaped as a spoon carved with the patterns of plant, which probably are some patterns trying to depict the sacrifice of " 社 " meaning the God of the land and his altar. The side is carved with a profile of an awing bird, and a small hole was gouged out at the reverse side for tying and hanging. The carved spoon is exquisite and delicate, and it must be a special daily utensil. It was unearthed in Zishan Ruins, Yuyao City, Zhejiang Province, in 1996.

Preserved in Institute of Cultural Relics and Archaeology of Zhejiang Province

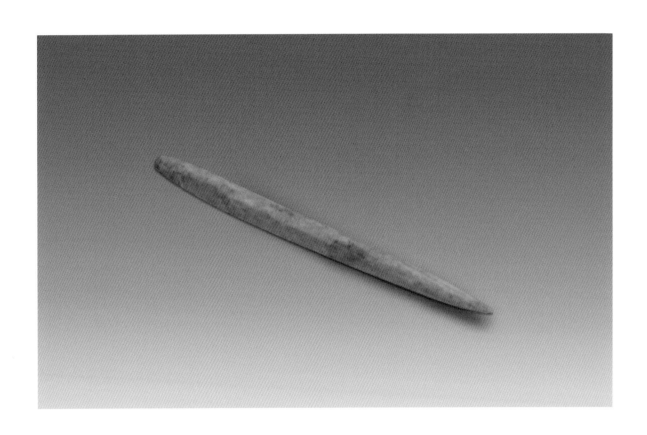

骨针

新石器时代，大溪文化

骨质

长 9.2 厘米

Bone Needle

Daxi Culture, the Neolithic Age

Bone

Length 9.2 cm

形体较小，一端较为尖利，而另一端稍残，亦为较原始的针刺工具。由原四川省文物管理委员会提供。

成都中医药大学中医药传统文化博物馆藏

The needle is small in size. It is relatively sharp at one end and deficient and blunt at the other. It's a primitive acupuncture tool and was provided by former Sichuan Provincial Committee for Cultural Relics.

Preserved in Museum of Traditional Chinese Medicine Culture, Chengdu University of Traditional Chinese Medicine

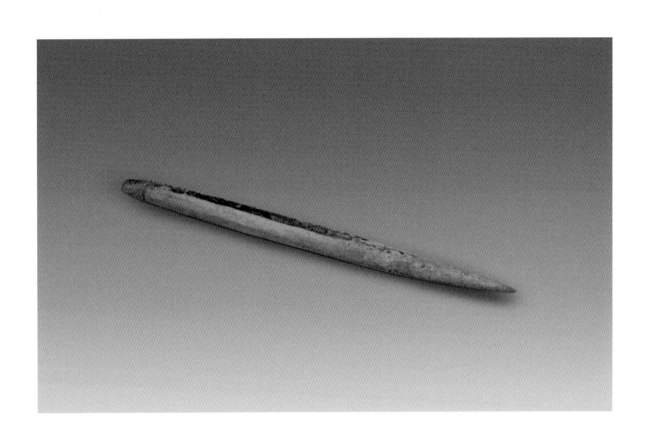

骨针

新石器时代，大溪文化

骨质

长 16 厘米

Bone Needle

Daxi Culture, the Neolithic Age

Bone

Length 16 cm

一端尖利，而另一端较圆钝，针体前部呈锥
形，便于手握，为较原始的针刺工具。由原
四川省文物管理委员会提供。

成都中医药大学中医药传统文化博物馆藏

The needle is a primitive acupuncture tool with
one end sharp and the other end blunt. The front
part of the needle is cone-shaped so that it is
easy to hold. It was provided by former Sichuan
Provincial Committee for Cultural Relics.
Preserved in Museum of Traditional Chinese
Medicine Culture, Chengdu University of Traditional
Chinese Medicine

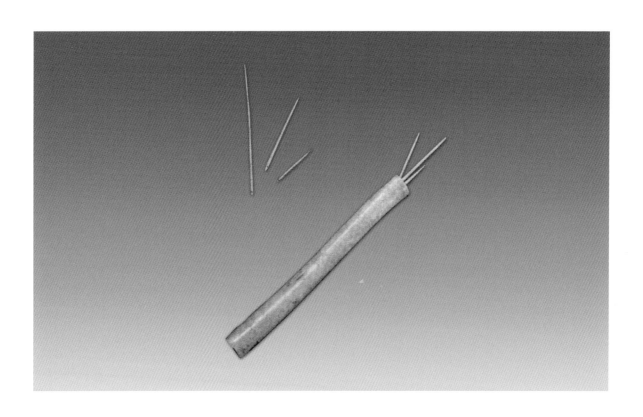

骨针（附针筒）

新石器时代，距今 5000 多年

骨质

针：最长 10.5 厘米，最短 3.8 厘米

针筒：长 15.3 厘米

Bone Needles (with Needle Container)

The Neolithic Age (5000 years ago)

Bone

Needles: Maximum Length 10.5 cm/Minimum Length 3.8 cm

Needle Container: Length 15.3 cm

用动物肢骨加工而成。骨针筒筒身光滑无纹饰，骨针分圆桯和肩桯两种，针尖尖锐，针身光滑，针孔清楚。1980 年内蒙古包头东郊出土。

内蒙古包头博物馆藏

The needles and the container were made of animal's limb bones. The container has a smooth body part without any decorations and inscriptions. The needles are of two types, the round ones and flat ones. Each one has a smooth body part, with one sharp end, and one end with clear needle-eye. The collections were unearthed in the eastern suburbs of Baotou City, Inner Mongolia, in 1980.

Preserved in Inner Mongolia Baotou Museum

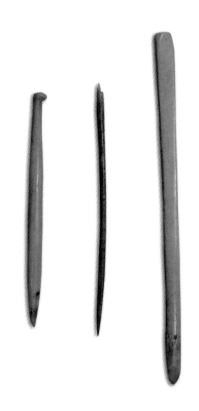

骨针

新石器时代

骨质

左：长 10.9 厘米，直径 0.5 厘米

中：长 7.2 厘米，直径 0.3 厘米

右：长 7.8 厘米，直径 1 厘米

Bone Needles

The Neolithic Age

Bone

The Left One: Length 10.9 cm/ Diameter 0.5 cm

The Middle One: Length 7.2 cm/ Diameter 0.3 cm

The Right One: Length 7.8 cm/ Diameter 1 cm

新石器时代骨质针具，为新石器时代早期先民用动物及人类骸骨所制作的针类医用工具，主要用于点刺患处。新石器时代早期对于穴位并没有明确的标定形式，他们只是通过生活经验认识到按压某个位置会对病痛有所缓解，而早期先民又认为动物及人类骸骨有驱邪扶正功能，故而以骨为材料制作驱除病痛器具。

张雅宗藏

The bone needles in the Neolithic age were the medical instruments made of animal or human bones by the earlier primitive people and were utilized in pricking method. In the earlier Neolithic Age, there was no clear systematic knowledge of acupuncture points, and people only learned from the daily experiences that pressing a certain spot on human body could relieve the painfulness caused by some diseases. The primitive people also thought that animal or human bones could get rid of the evil spirits, so bones were chosen as materials making instruments which could treat sickness and pains.

Collected by Zhang Yazong

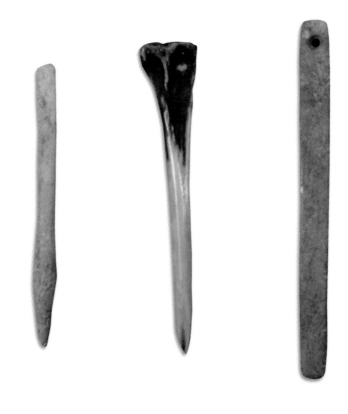

骨针刀

新石器时代

骨质

左：长 10.2 厘米，宽 0.8 厘米

中：长 8.8 厘米，宽 0.5 厘米

右：长 8.5 厘米，宽 0.3 厘米

Bone Needles and Knife

The Neolithic Age

Bone

The Left One: Length 10.2 cm/ Width 0.8 cm

The Middle One: Length 8.8 cm/ Width 0.5 cm

The Right One: Length 8.5 cm/ Width 0.3 cm

新石器时代骨质针刀器，一套三枚。从左至右，第一枚为骨针，尖状，主要用于刺压点按患处。第二枚为骨针按压器具，主要用于按压穴位与经络治疗。第三枚为骨质切割器，主要用于放血。早期医用工具特征明显，成序列。

张雅宗藏

The three pieces bone needles and knives are a set. The one on the left is a bone needle with a pointed end which could be used to puncture the affected spots on human body. The one in the middle is a pressing tool, mainly for pressing acupuncture points and treating meridian systems. And The Right One is a bone knife used as a cutting tool for bloodletting. The collection has the characteristics of earlier medical instruments in a series.

Collected by Zhang Yazong

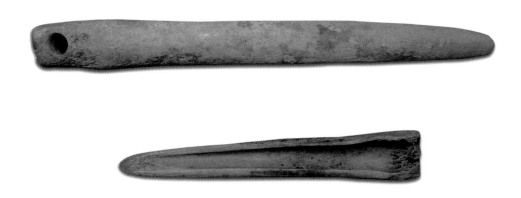

骨刀

新石器时代

骨质

上：长 18.8 厘米，宽 1.8 厘米

下：长 12 厘米，宽 1.4 厘米

Bone Knives

The Neolithic Age

Bone

The Upper One: Length 18.8 cm/ Width 1.8 cm

The Lower One: Length 12 cm/ Width 1.4 cm

骨质刀具，是中医起源阶段出现最早的刀形
器具之一。

张雅宗藏

The bone cutting tools are one of the earliest
knife tools in the stage of traditional Chinese
medicine origin.

Collected by Zhang Yazong

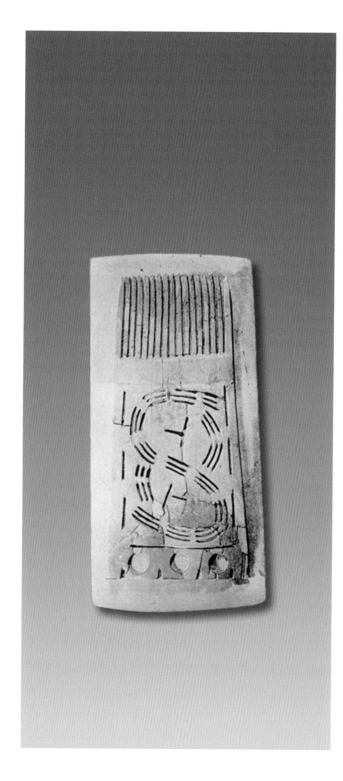

缕空回旋纹象牙梳

新石器时代（距今 5000 年左右）

象牙质

长 16.4 厘米，宽 8 厘米

Ivory Comb with Circle Round Designs in Open-work

The Neolithic Age (about 5000 years ago)

Ivory

Length 16.4 cm/ Width 8 cm

背厚齿薄，顶端有四个楔形开口，其下镂刻三个圆孔，梳身中部用平行三行条孔组成类"8"字形镂空装饰内填"T"字纹。梳端及左右两侧各刻有两三个条孔，构成一个长方形装饰面。下端十六个细密的梳齿，保存完好。可用于梳理头发。为现知中国最早的象牙雕梳。1959年山东泰安大汶口出土。

中国国家博物馆藏

The comb has thick back and thin teeth, with four wedge-shaped openings on the top, and three round holes carved in open-work underneath. The middle part is carved with 3 paralleled slot holes which formed a shape similar to "8" with "T" patterns carved in middle. Three or two slot holes are carved on the end and two sides of the comb, forming rectangular decorations. The comb has 16 fine and close comb teeth and is preserved in good condition. It can be used to comb hair. So far, the collection is known as the earliest ivory-carving comb in China. It was unearthed in Dawenkou, Tai'an City, Shandong Province, in 1959.

Preserved in National Museum of China

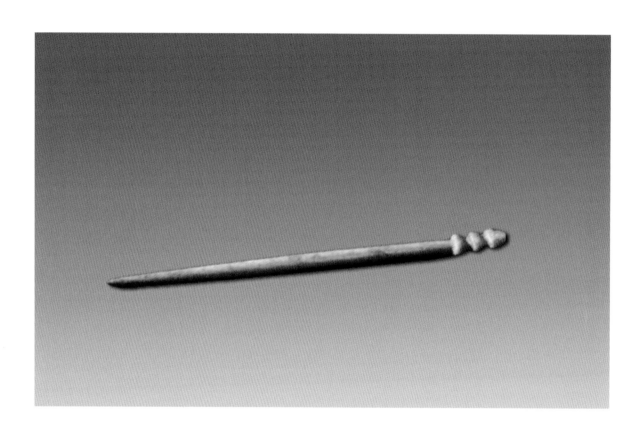

骨簪

新石器时代

骨质

长 14.5 厘米

Bone Hairpin

The Neolithic Age

Bone

Length 14.5 cm

簪身平滑，尖端圆钝，上端雕磨成三节似蘑菇塔状，颈部较细，中间稍粗。1978年昌都卡若遗址出土。

西藏博物馆藏

The hairpin has a smooth body part with one round and blunt end and one end made in three mushroom-like shapes. The neck part is relatively slim and the middle part thick. The collection was unearthed in Kano Ruins, Changdu City, Tibet, in 1978.

Preserved in Tibet Museum

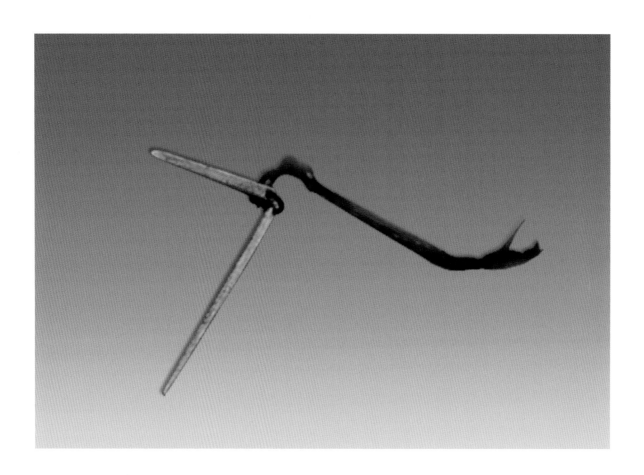

骨针

新石器时代晚期
骨质
长 4.2 厘米

Bone Needles

The Late Neolithic Age

Bone

Length 4.2 cm

针孔圆滑，针身笔直，制作精细，是人类早
期的缝纫工具，又能应用于医疗。1978 年昌
都卡若遗址出土。

西藏博物馆藏

The collection is of fine craftsmanship, with
perfectly straight body part and a smooth and
round needle-eye on one end. It used to be a
sewing tool as well as a medical instrument for
primitive people. The needle was unearthed in
Kano Ruins, Changdu City, Tibet, in 1978.
Preserved in Tibet Museum

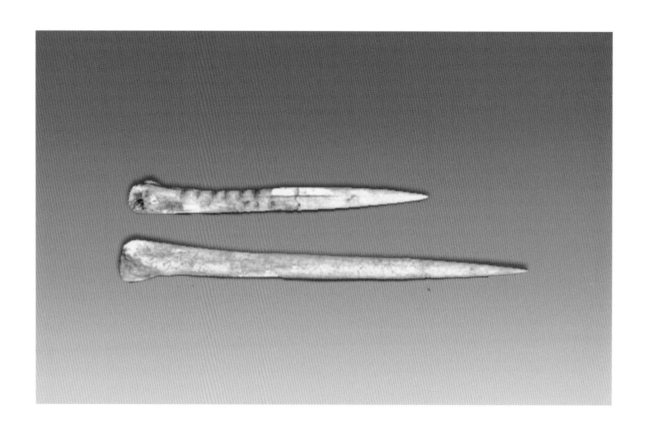

骨锥

新石器时代晚期

骨质

最长 17 厘米

Bone Awls

The Late Neolithic Age

Bone

Length of the Longer Awl 17 cm

制作精细，表面光滑，锥尖锋利。1978 年昌

都卡若遗址出土。

西藏博物馆藏

The collections are well made, with smooth
body parts and sharp ends, which can be used
as tools in daily life and work, sometimes as
acupuncture tools in treatment. The bone awls
were unearthed in Kano Ruins, Changdu City,
Tibet, in 1978.

Preserved in Tibet Museum

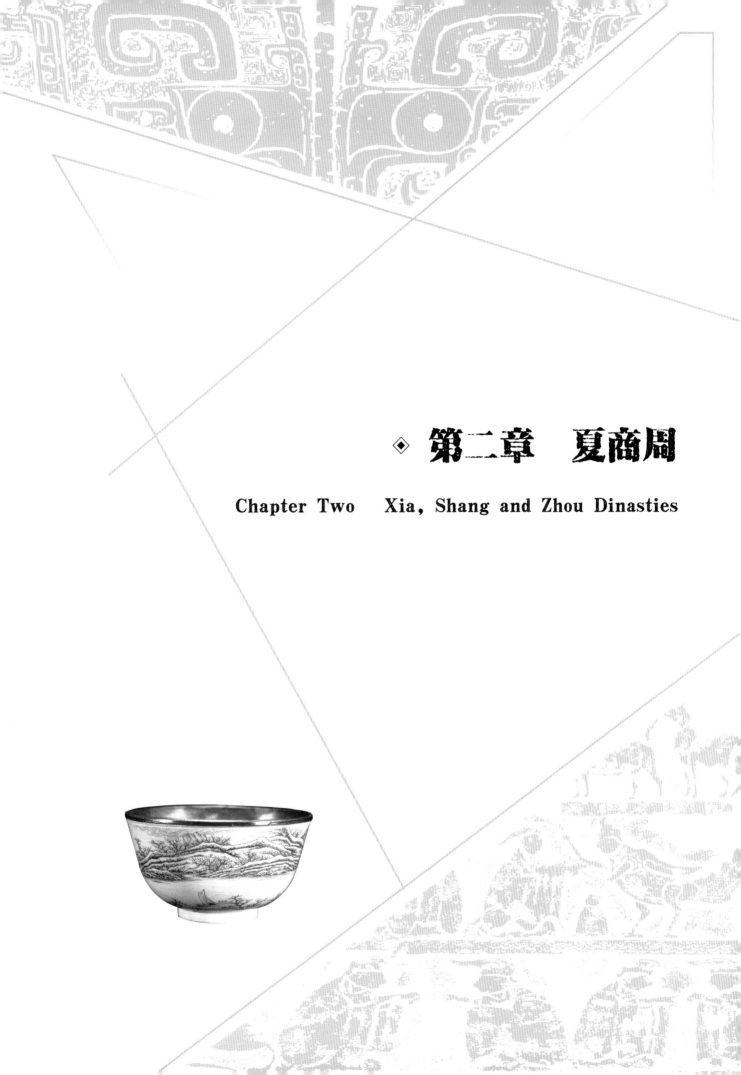

◇ 第二章　夏商周

Chapter Two　Xia, Shang and Zhou Dinasties

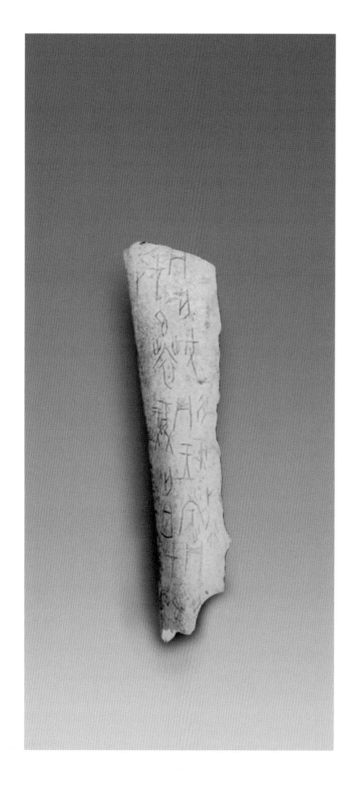

甲骨

商

骨质

长 7.5 厘米，宽 1.7 厘米

Oracle Bone

Shang Dynasty

Bone

Length 7.5 cm/ Width 1.7 cm

正面刻辞 3 条，计 21 字，均是占卜前的贞辞；

背面有灼烧痕。

山西博物院藏

The obverse side of the bone is engraved with three lines of inscriptions. There are a total of 21 faithful words before divination. There are burn marks on the reverse side.

Preserved in Shanxi Museum

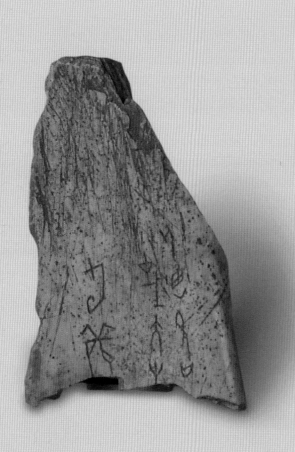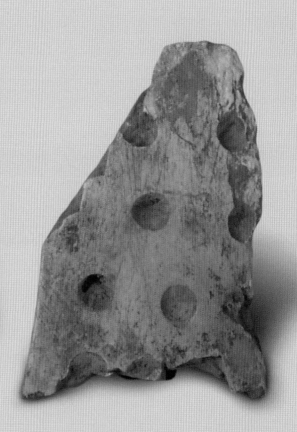

甲骨片

商

骨质

长 8.6 厘米，宽 5.7 厘米

近三角形块状，为甲骨。该甲骨一面刻有文
字（待考），一面有钻孔，可能用于占卜。
1964 年入藏。保存基本完好。

中华医学会 / 上海中医药大学医史博物馆藏

Oracle Bone Piece

Shang Dynasty

Bone

Length 8.6 cm/ Width 5.7 cm

This oracle bone is almost triangular in shape,
with some words inscribed on one side and
holes drilled on the other. They might be
utilized for divination. It was collected in 1964
and is still in good condition.

Preserved in Chinese Medical Association/
Museum of Chinese Medicine, Shanghai
University of Traditional Chinese Medicine

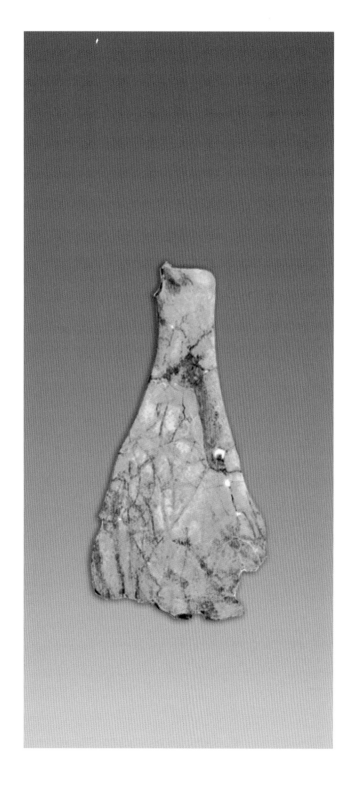

卜骨

西周

骨质

长 39 厘米，宽 22 厘米

Divining Bone

West Zhou Dynasty

Bone

Length 39 cm/ Width 22 cm

为牛肩胛骨制成。正面钻窝处有许多小兆；两面周边均经打磨；背面近骨臼处有钻窝 16 个，不规则地排列；距右边 1 厘米处有刻辞一行 8 字，初释为"北宫口三止（趾）又（有）疾贞"。

山西博物院藏

The bone is a cow's shoulder blade. There are many small omens near the drilled dents on the obverse side. The rims of both sides of the bone were polished. On the reverse side, there are 16 drilled dents near the bone socket, which are in irregular order. A line of eight ancient Chinese characters was engraved about 1 cm to the right side.

Preserved in Shanxi Museum

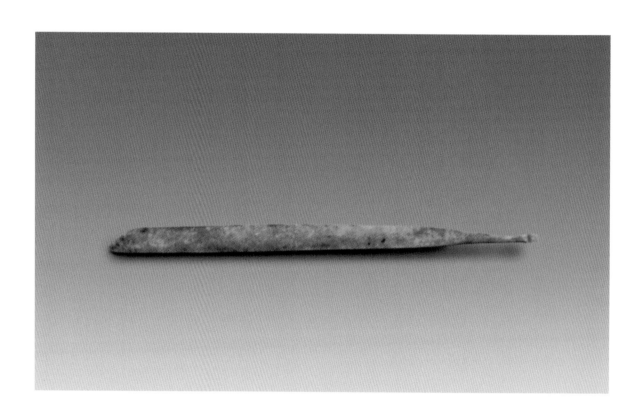

挖耳勺

西周

骨质

残长 10.3 厘米，勺径 0.4 厘米

Earpick

West Zhou Dynasty

Bone

Remnant Length 10.3 cm/ Diameter 0.4 cm

细长柄，柄的一端制出一个小勺，是一种用

于掏挖耵聍的工具。

宝鸡市周原博物馆藏

The collection has a long and slim handle, with

one end shaped in form of a little spoon. It was

used as a tool to clean ears.

Preserved in Zhouyuan Museum of Baoji City

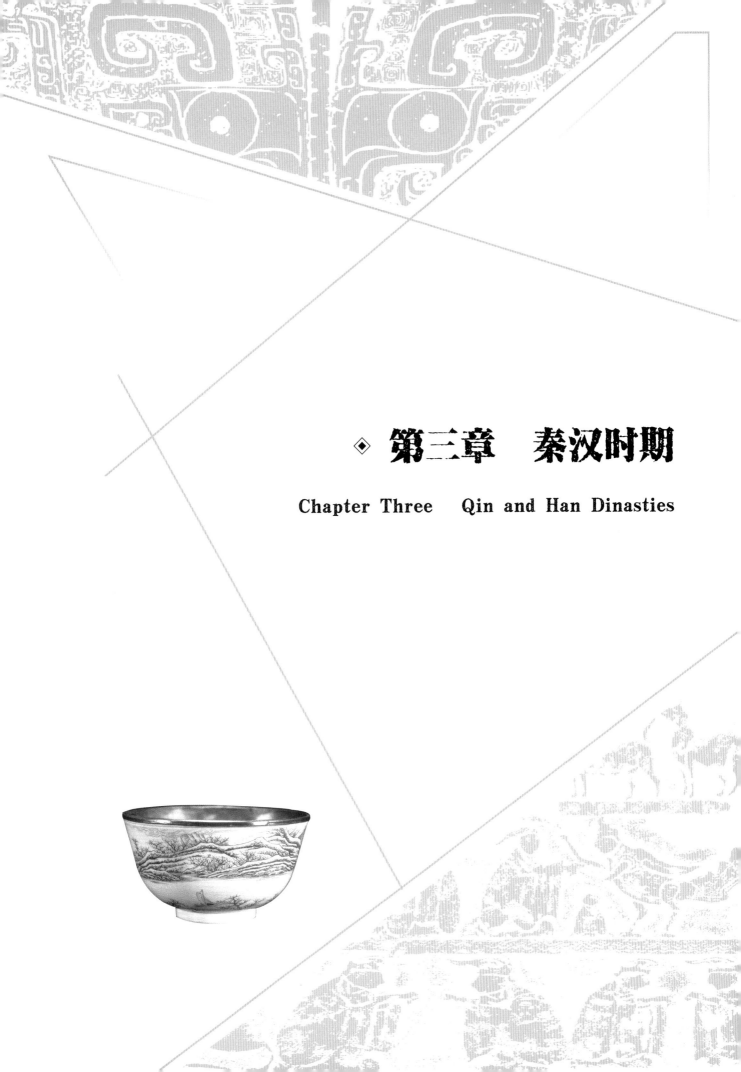

◇ 第三章 秦汉时期

Chapter Three Qin and Han Dinasties

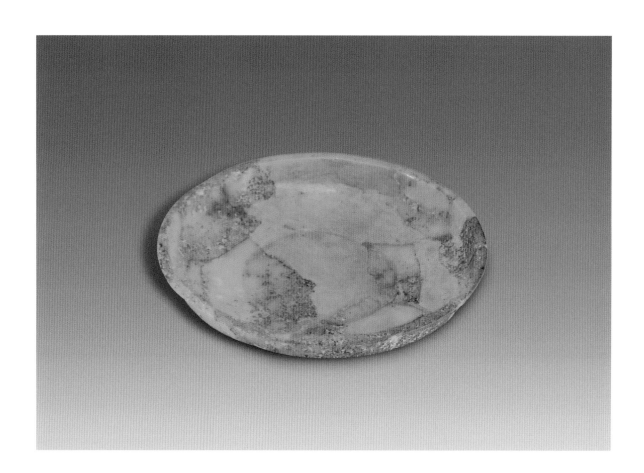

玻璃盘

西汉

玻璃质

口径 19.7 厘米，高 3.2 厘米

Glass Plate

Western Han Dynasty

Glass

Mouth Diameter 19.7 cm/ Height 3.2 cm

盘侈口，平折沿，浅腹折收，平底。湖绿色，半透明，光润如玉。破口处折射玻璃光，经光谱定性分析，主要成分是硅和铅，并含有钠和钡。采用模铸成型工艺，通体抛光，制作精美，对研究我国早期玻璃器的制造具有重要价值。

河北博物院藏

The plate has a wide opening, a folded rim, a contracted shallow belly and a flat bottom. The translucent light green plate is as smooth as jade. Lights are reflected from crevasse on the plate. The spectrum analysis shows that the main components of the glass are silicon and lead including some sodium and barium. The entire plate is polished exquisitely through the process of die casting and forming. It is of great value for studying and researching the glassmaking in the early stage in China.

Preserved in Hebei Museum

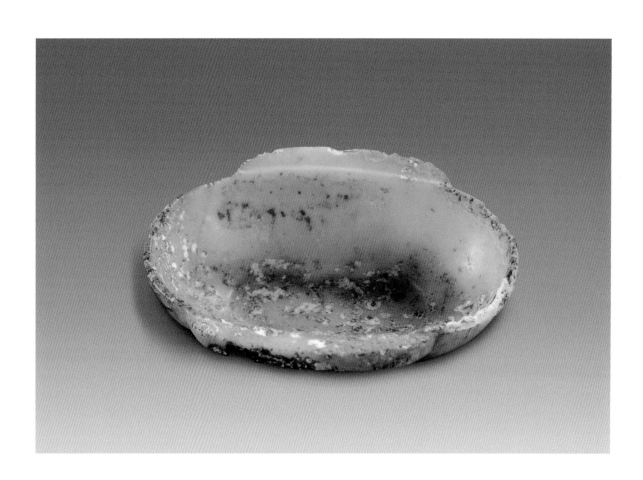

玻璃耳杯

西汉

玻璃质

长 13.5 厘米，宽 10.4 厘米，高 3.4 厘米

Eared Glass Cup

Western Han Dynasty

Glass

Length 13.5 cm/ Width 10.4 cm/ Height 3.4 cm

椭圆形，两侧有耳微向上翘，假圈足。湖绿色，半透明，光润如玉。破口处射玻璃光，经光谱定性分析，主要成分是硅和铅，并含有钠和钡。采用模铸成型工艺，通体抛光，制作精美，对研究我国早期玻璃器的制造具有重要价值。

河北博物院藏

The oval cup has two upturned ears on its two sides and a fake foot ring. The translucent light green cup is as smooth as jade. Lights are reflected from crevasses on the cup. The spectrum analysis shows that the main components of the glass are silicium and lead including some sodium and barium. The entire cup is polished exquisitely through the process of die casting and forming. It is of great value for studying and researching the glassmaking in the early stage in China.

Preserved in Hebei Museum

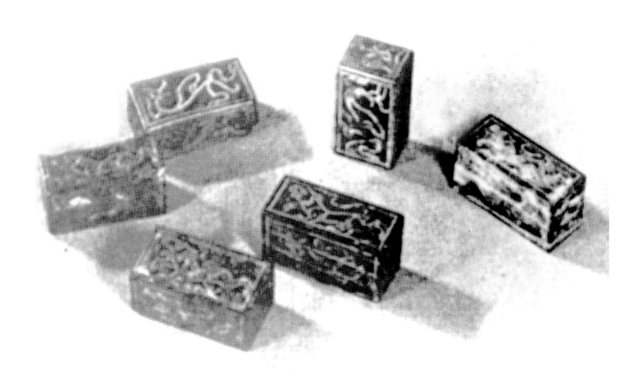

六博棋子

西汉

象牙质

长 3.1 厘米，宽 1.5 厘米，厚 1.2 厘米

Pieces of Traditional Chess Game (Liubo Chess Pieces)

Western Han

Ivory

Length 3.1 cm/ Width1.5 cm/ Thickness 1.2 cm

共出土 8 枚，大小一致，边缘有阴刻的直线
为框，其中 4 枚的六面框内有阴刻龙纹，另
外 4 枚的六面框内有阴刻奔虎。雕工精巧，
形象生动。1974 年北京市大葆台 1 号西汉墓
出土。

北京大葆台西汉墓博物馆藏

There are eight pieces in total. They are of the
same size. The straight lines in intaglio along
the rims are used as their frames. Four of them
are carved with dragon patterns within their six
frames and the other four running tigers, and all
of the patterns are in intaglio. The carved pieces
are exquisite and delicate with vivid images.
They were unearthed in No. 1 of Western Han
Tomb in Dabaotai, Beijing, in 1974.
Presered in Beijing Dabaotai Museum of West
Han Dynasty

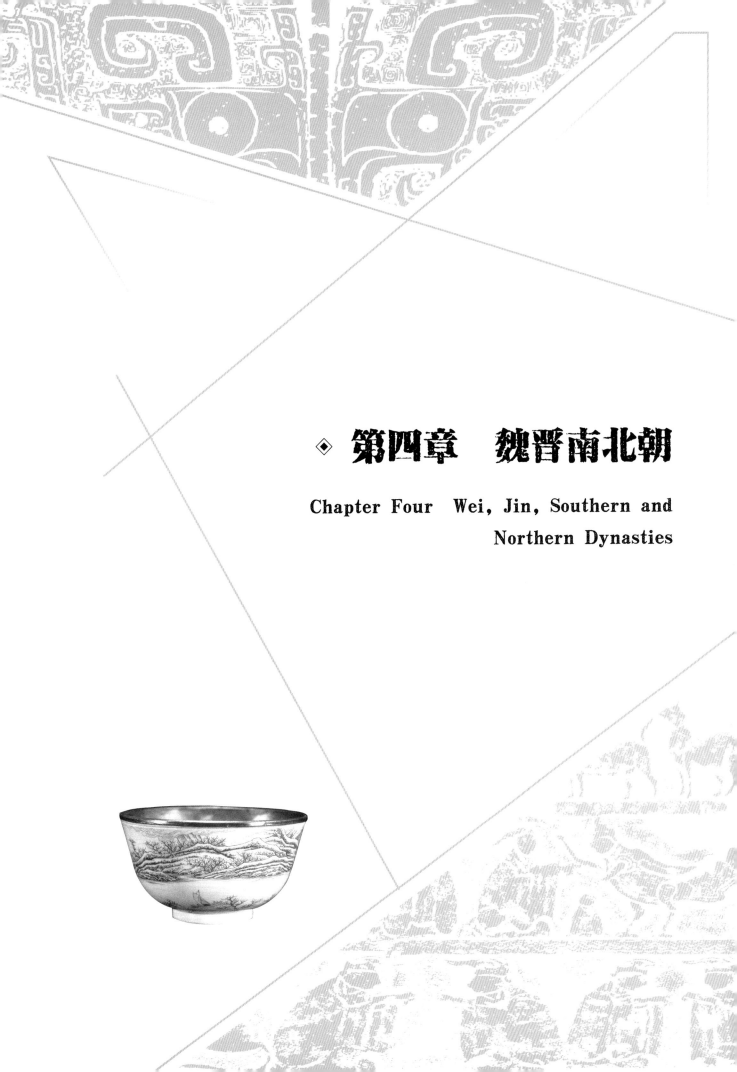

◇ 第四章　魏晋南北朝

Chapter Four　Wei, Jin, Southern and
Northern Dynasties

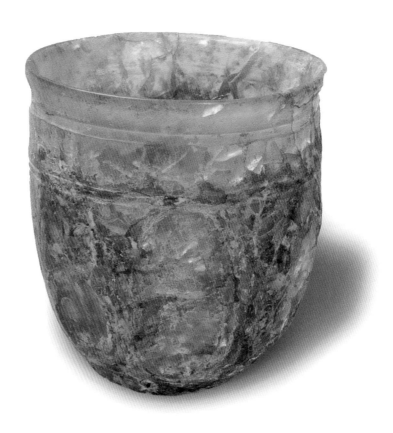

玻璃杯

东晋

玻璃质

口径 9.6 厘米，底径 2.5 厘米，高 10.4 厘米

玻璃白色中呈黄绿色，较透明，内有气泡，因长期受水土浸蚀，表面有银白色的风化层。杯呈直桶形，圆口稍外侈，平底略凹。口沿外上下刻一周弦纹，中间底部为较瘦长的花瓣纹，表面平滑。此件玻璃杯是这一时期出土文物中极为罕见的珍品，在当时则被视为"宝器"，从其造型及工艺手法看，为舶来品，它是六朝时期我国与外国物质文化交流的重要例证。出土于东晋丞相王导家族的墓葬。

南京市博物馆藏

Glass

Eastern Jin Dynasty

Glass

Mouth Diameter 9.6 cm/ Bottom Diameter 2.5 cm/ Height 10.4 cm

The glass is white in yellow green, comparatively transparent and has bubbles inside. Because of long-time erosion by water and soil, there is a silver white weathered layer on the surface. The barrel-shaped glass has a round mouth which is slightly flared outward. The bottom is flat and little concave. With a smooth surface, the cup is carved with a bow string pattern up and down along the outer rim of the mouth and a long thin flower petal pattern at the lower part of the glass. This glass was extremely rare among the historic relics unearthed at that time and was regarded as a rare and precious treasure in those days. It was an imported product according to its shape, techniques and craftsmanship, and was a very important example of cultural and business exchanges in the period of the Six Dynasties. It was unearthed from the tombs of Wang Dao's family, one of the prime ministers in the Eastern Jin Dynasty.

Preserved in Nanjing Museum

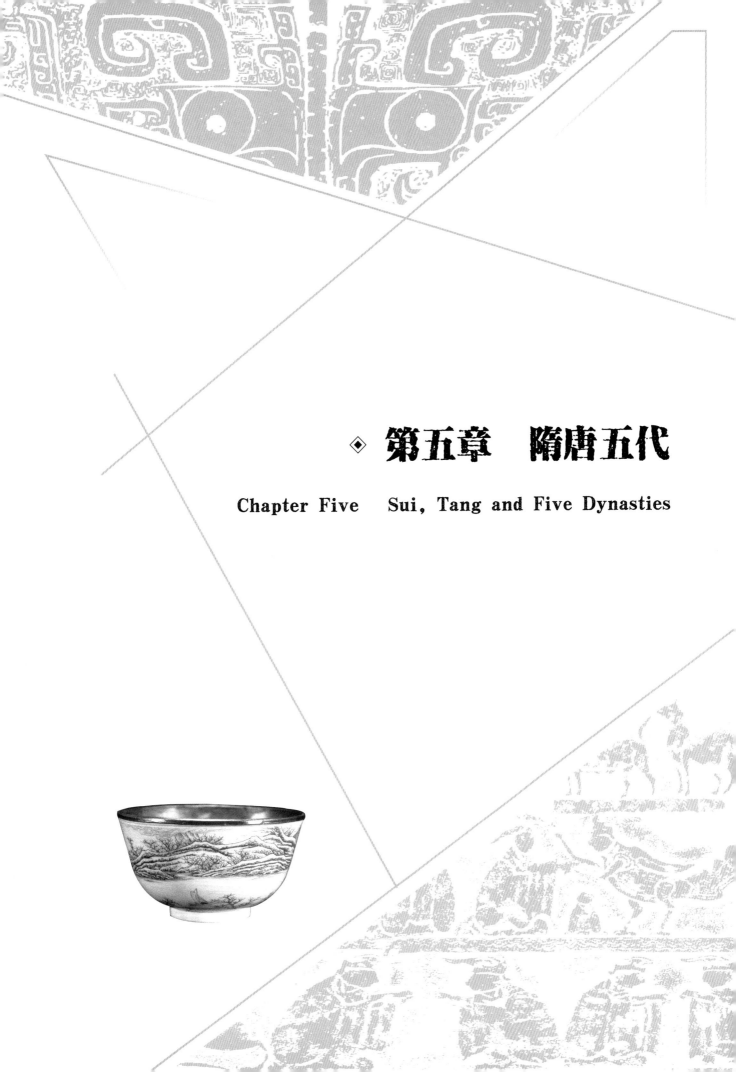

◇ 第五章　隋唐五代

Chapter Five　Sui, Tang and Five Dynasties

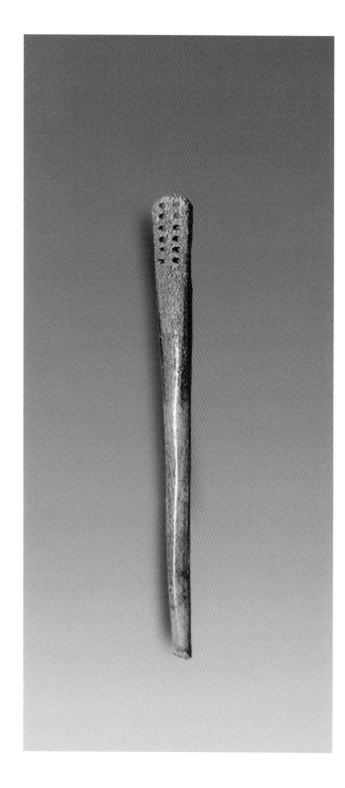

牙刷柄

唐

骨质

长 17.8 厘米，头部宽 1.1 厘米，孔径 0.3 厘米

Toothbrush Handle

Tang Dynasty

Bone

Length 17.8 cm/ Head Width 1.1 cm/ Hole Diameter 0.3 cm

共出土 4 把，刷毛已全部脱落。 此柄前端植
毛部共 12 孔，两排，孔内上下相通。1985 年
成都市指挥街遗址出土。

　　成都中医药大学中医药传统文化博物馆藏

The hair of the four unearthed toothbrush
handles has completely come off. There are
12 holes in two rows at the front end of the
handle which are for fixing hair. The holes are
interlinked up and down. They were unearthed
in Zhihui Street Site, Chengdu City, in 1985.
Preserved in Museum of Traditional Chinese
Medicine Culture, Chengdu University of Traditional
Chinese Medicine

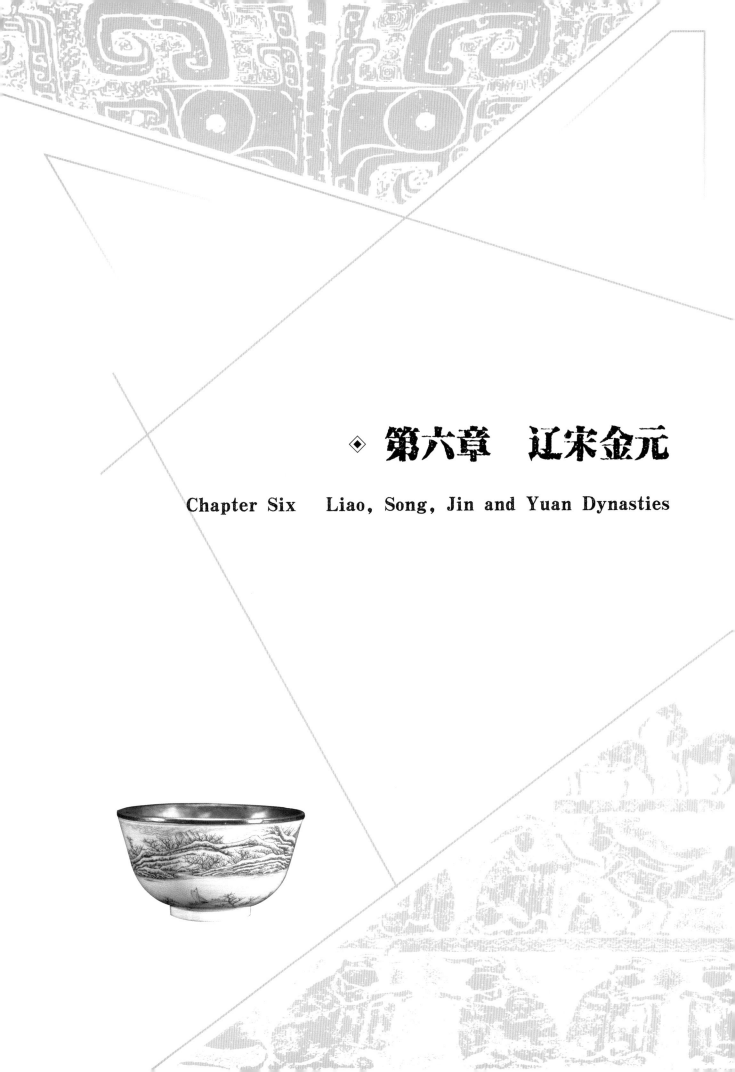

◇ 第六章 辽宋金元

Chapter Six　　Liao, Song, Jin and Yuan Dynasties

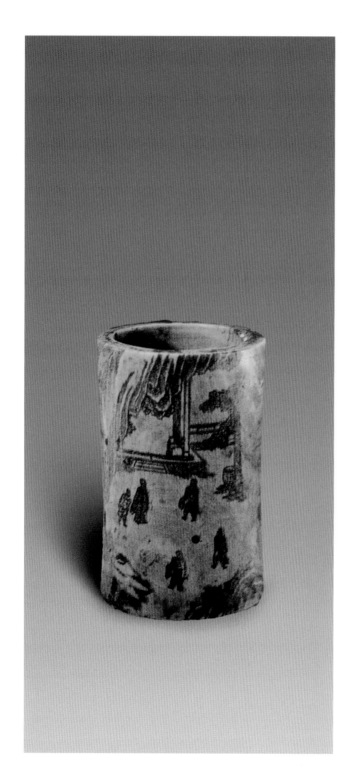

牙雕蹴鞠图笔筒

宋

象牙质

直径 10.9 厘米，高 16 厘米

Ivory Brush Holder Carved with Picture of Four Men Kicking the Ball (Cuju)

Song Dynasty

Ivory

Diameter 10.9 cm/ Height 16 cm

图案绘于笔筒的筒身。在一宽敞的庭院中，四个人正在相向蹴鞠，另一人侧立一旁，似为童仆。由画面中蹴鞠的形式看，应为宋代流行的以讲究技巧为特点的"白打"式蹴鞠。

安徽博物院藏

A picture is painted on the body of the brush holder. In a spacious courtyard, four men standing face to face are kicking the ball, and another one who seems to be a houseboy, is standing aside. Cu means to kick things, while ju is a leather ball filled with some materials. Cuju is a kind of traditional football game in China. The style of the Cuju in the picture might be Baida, one of the popular ways of kicking the ball in the Song Dynasty, meaning the player should use a lot of skills in playing.

Preserved in Anhui Museum

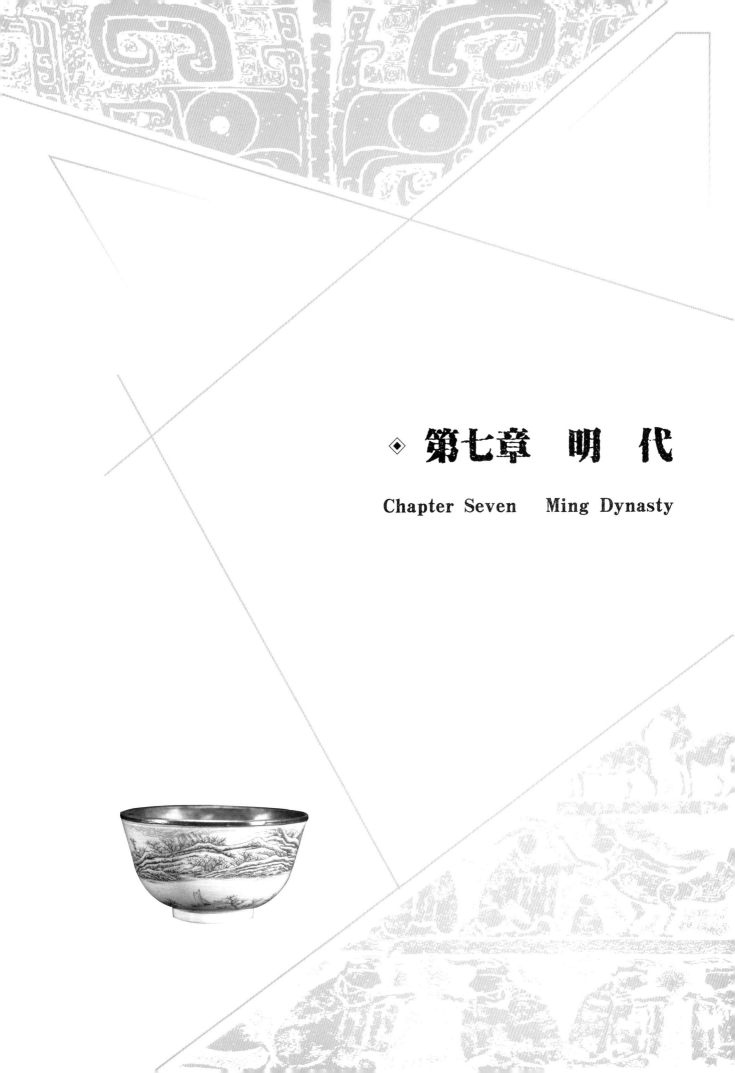

◆ 第七章 明 代

Chapter Seven　Ming Dynasty

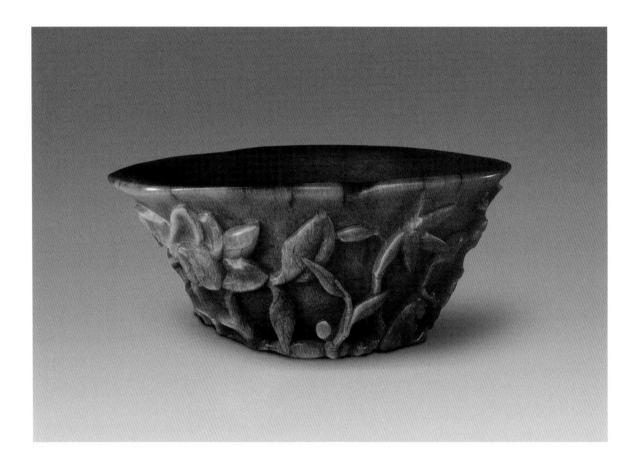

犀角雕花卉洗

明初

犀角质

口径 14.9 ～ 18.7 厘米，底径 8.9 ～ 9.1 厘米，高 8 厘米

Rhinoceros Horn Ware Carved with Flowers and Plants Design

Early Ming Dynasty

Rhinoceros Horn

Mouth Diameter 14.9-18.7 cm/ Bottom Diameter 8.9-9.1 cm/ Height 8 cm

以犀角近根部雕成。淡褐色，口如花瓣式，收腰，底为竹枝式圈足，并浅雕出一灵芝。杯身雕桃花、桃实、玉兰、竹叶等，浅刻叶脉、花筋。

故宫博物院藏

The light brown ware is carved out of the root segment of a horn. It has a petal-like mouth, a contracted waist and a foot ring in bamboo pole style which is engraved with a lucid ganoderma in high relief. The body is carved with peach flowers, peach fruit, Yulan magnolia and bamboo leaves, plus petal veins and leaf veins in bas-relief.

Preserved in The Palace Museum

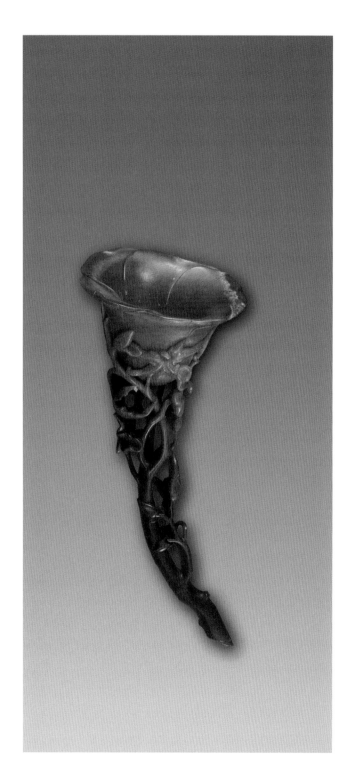

犀角雕蜀葵天然形杯

明初

犀角质

口径 11.8 ~ 14.6 厘米，高 39.7 厘米

Rhinoceros Horn Cup Carved with Hollyhock Design in Natural Shape

Early Ming Dynasty

Rhinoceros Horn

Mouth Diameter 11.8-14.6 cm/ Height 39.7 cm

以广角，即非洲犀角制成。随形镂雕作折枝蜀葵式，构思巧妙，主枝至腰处分裂为二，于杯口处合抱，又雕小枝盘绕其间，穿插转侧，变化多端。杯口之花瓣形，随犀角纹路呈螺旋式，杯底挖出花蕊。

故宫博物院藏

The cup is made of African rhinoceros horn and carved into the shape of a hollyhock in open work with clever conception and design. The main branch at the waist place is divided into two parts which then fold together again at the cup mouth. Some carved small branches are entwining the main branch. The petal shape mouth is carved in spiral way according to the texture of the rhinoceros horn. The bottom of the cup is hollowly engraved into buds of the hollyhock.

Preserved in The Palace Museum

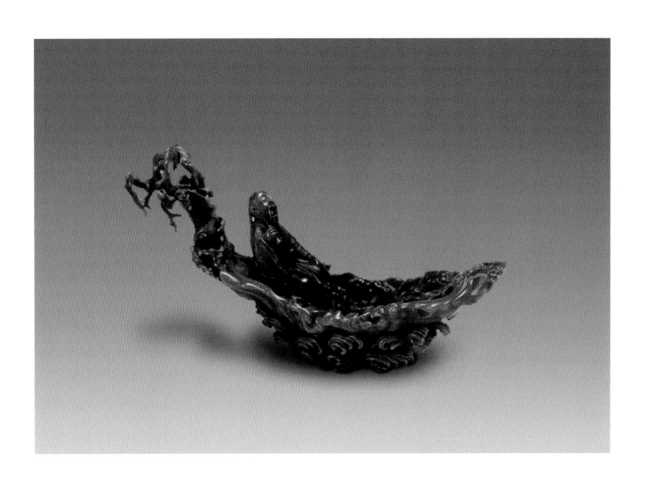

犀角仙人乘搓

明末

犀角质

长 21.1 厘米，宽 6.6 厘米，高 11.1 厘米

Rhinoceros Horn Ware Carved with Immortal Design

Late Ming Dynasty

Rhinoceros Horn

Length 21.1 cm/ Width 6.6 cm/ Height 11.1 cm

长形，浅栗色。采用圆雕、浮雕等技法，将犀角制成内中空、瘿节累累的枯树形舟。舟首浅平，舟尾枯枝翘起，一长髯老人，身着长衫，头戴素巾，手持经卷，面带微笑端坐于槎中。舟下水波翻涌成漩，似在激流中航行。

故宫博物院藏

The collection has a long shape and light chestnut color. The rhinoceros horn is engraved hollowly inside and made into a shape of a raft with withered tree burls by the skills of embossment and circular engravure. The prow is shallow and flat while the stern is warping upward. With the sutra in his hand, an old man who has long beard and wears long gown and plain scarf is sitting on the raft with a smile. Underneath the raft is the wave rolling over and over into whirlpool just as the raft is sailing in vehement turbulence.

Preserved in The Palace Museum

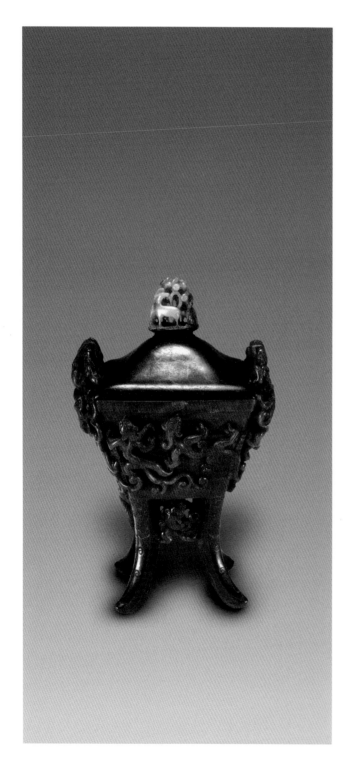

犀角镂雕蟠螭双耳四足鼎

明末

犀角质

口径 7.9 ~ 9.5 厘米，足径 6.4 ~ 8.6 厘米，

通高 21 厘米

Four-footed Rhinoceros Horn Wine Cup Carved with Two Interlaced Hydra Ears

Late Ming Dynasty

Rhinoceros Horn

Mouth Diameter 7.9–9.5 cm/ Foot Diameter 6.4–8.6cm/ Height 21 cm

亚洲犀牛额前角制成。仿古方鼎形，四撇足。以浮雕技法将方鼎耳刻成堆垒如云的螭纹朝天耳，又将犀角尖切劈的四足用热烫技法向外弯撇。在鼎壁浅刻勾云如意纹锦地上，共有15条大小蟠螭攀附，一条苍龙潜伏于底足之间，龙腾螭跃，活灵活现。鼎上配有嵌鹿鹤灵芝纹及白玉钮的红木盖。

故宫博物院藏

The cup is made of the forehead horn of Asian rhinoceros. It is in the style of ancient squared Ding-vessel with four flared feet. The upturned ears are carved in relief into paste-on-paste cloud-like hydra patterns. The four feet cut from the horn sharp is made outward and flared with the skills of heat shocking. Fifteen different sizes of hydras are clinging to the wall of the cup with cloud and Ruyi patterns in shallow carving. A dragon is lurking among the four feet of the bottom. The flying dragons and hydras are vividly depicted. The cup has a redwood lid with a white jade knob inlaid with the patterns of deers, cranes and ganoderma.

Preserved in The Palace Museum

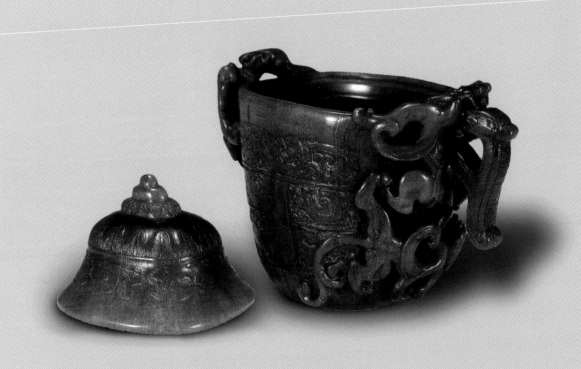

鲍天成款犀角雕双螭耳仿古螭虎纹执壶

明末

犀角质

口径 7.8 ~ 15 厘米，高 13 厘米

采用镂刻、圆雕技法，用两个亚洲犀角合并制成带流执壶。一个小犀角为盖，一个大犀角为壶身。壶盖形如盔帽，色比较深，饰蕉叶纹，盖上饰回纹钮，为后嵌。壶身左侧为光素流，一条螭从壶身攀绕着向流口瞪视。右边为柄，三条螭围绕着柄把上下腾戏。壶身纹饰从底向上为蕉叶纹、兽面、蟠螭纹。

故宫博物院藏

Rhinoceros Horn Ewer with Dragon Shaped Handles Carved by Bao Tiancheng

Late Ming Dynasty

Rhinoceros Horn

Mouth Diameter 7.8-15 cm/ Height 13 cm

The ewer with a spout is made with two Asian rhinoceros horns with the skills of openwork and circular engravure. The little horn is made into a lid while the big one is made into the body of the ewer. The lid is shaped as a helmet which has dark color, and is decorated with the patterns of banana leaves. The knob with a kind of pattern which looks like the Chinese character "Hui" is inlaid afterwards. The left side of the ewer is a spout with no decoration and a hydra is clinging to the body and staring at the spout. The right side is a handle with three hydras flying and playing around it. From the bottom to the top, the body is decorated with patterns of banana leaves, animal faces and hydra and tiger designs.

Preserved in The Palace Museum

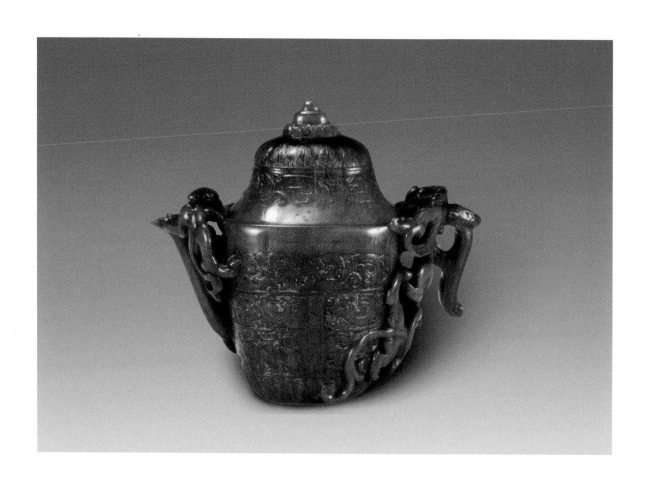

鲍天成款犀角雕双螭耳仿古执壶

明末

犀角质

长 15 厘米，宽 7.8 厘米，高 13 厘米

Rhinoceros Horn Ewer with Dragon Shaped Handles Carved by Bao Tiancheng

Late Ming Dynasty

Rhinoceros Horn

Length 15 cm/ Width 7.8 cm/ Height 13 cm

雕刻艺人采用镂刻圆雕枝法，以两个亚洲犀角合并制成带流执壶。小犀角为壶盖，大犀角为壶身，壳盖形如盔帽，色较深，刻回文钮，为后嵌，盖周刻蕉叶纹。1985 年叶义捐献。

故宫博物院藏

The ewer with a spout is made with two Asian rhinoceros horns with the skills of openwork and circular engravure. The little horn is made into a lid while the big one is made into the body of the ewer. The lid is shaped as a helmet which has dark color and is decorated with the patterns of banana leaves. The knob with a kind of pattern which looks like the Chinese character "Hui" is inlaid afterwards. It was donated by Ye Yi, in 1985.

Preserved in The Palace Museum

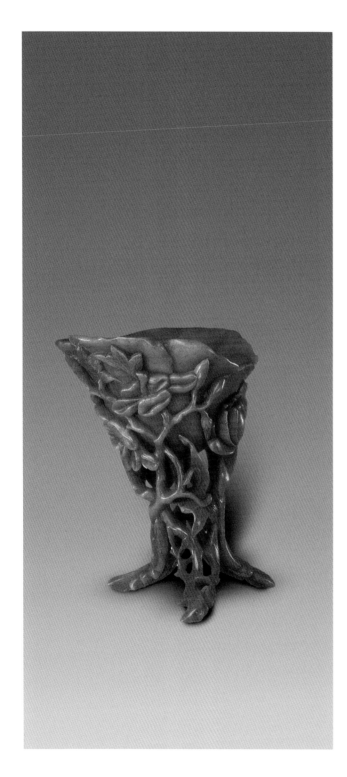

犀角雕花三足觥

明末

犀角质

口径 14 厘米，足径 11.4 厘米，高 16.9 厘米

Tri-footed Rhinoceros Horn Wine Vessel Carved with Flowers

Late Ming Dynasty

Rhinoceros Horn

Mouth Diameter 14 cm/ Foot Diameter 11.4 cm/

Height 16.9 cm

如一大朵盛开的花，三足如三束折枝花果，枝蔓交错，托抱觥体。雕镂荷花、海棠、蜀葵、荔枝等，将其枝叶、花朵的开阖、仰俯、向背、转侧、叠压、穿插等进行悉心的组织，尤其是镂雕工艺的熟练应用，无疑拓展了犀角雕刻的表现力，使观者在不知不觉中忘记了犀角本来的形状。

故宫博物院藏

The vessel looks like a big fully blooming flower. The three feet look like three branches with flowers and fruits which are intricate and twisted, supporting and half embracing the body. It is carved with lotus, cherry-apple tree, hollyhock, and litchi in open work. The sculptor carefully arranged the branches and flowers, by making them in various styles. The proficient and skillful applications of the openwork undoubtedly develop the expressive force of rhinoceros horn carvings which also make appreciators unconsciously forget about the original form of the rhinoceros horn.

Preserved in The Palace Museum

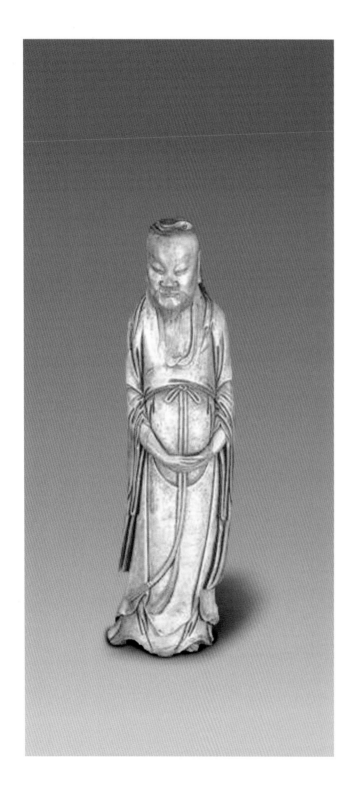

象牙雕老人

明末

象牙质

底径 6.5 ～ 8.3 厘米，高 9.8 厘米

Ivory Statue of Old Man

Late Ming Dynasty

Ivory

Bottom Diameter 6.5-8.3 cm/ Height 9.8 cm

随小象牙自然弯曲形状，以圆雕技法刻一老人裸臂赤足，头戴幞巾，身着广袖长衫，双手交叉在腹前，腰束丝绳，双眼微眯，头微低，下视前方，一派隐士风度。

故宫博物院藏

The statue is carved into an old man's shape according to the natural curving form of a small ivory by the skills of circular engravure. The carved old man has naked arms and bare feet. He is wearing a long gown with wide sleeves, a silk braid around waist and a scarf on the head. With his head slightly down, eyes squinting and looking down at the place ahead, he crosses his hands in front of his belly with hermit demeanour.

Preserved in The Palace Museum

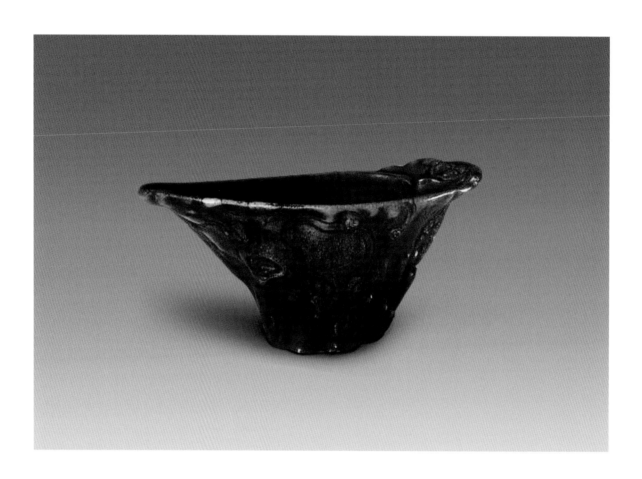

犀角雕富贵万代杯

明末

犀角质

口径 9.9 ~ 17.3 厘米，足径 4.3 ~ 6 厘米，高 7.6 厘米

Rhinoceros Horn Cup with Motif of Being Rich and Honourable for Generations

Late Ming Dynasty

Rhinoceros Horn

Mouth Diameter 9.9–17.3 cm/ Foot Diameter 4.3–6 cm/ Height 7.6 cm

杯造型以角形为基础，广口，敛腹，俯视呈椭圆形，杯口一侧弧线较长，如流状，另一侧则于口沿处雕镂瘿形纹饰。

故宫博物院藏

The cup is in the natural form of the rhinoceros horn. It has a wide opening and a contracted belly. The mouth is oval-shaped when overlooked. The arc on the one side of the mouth is longer just like a spout and the other side is carved with gall-shaped patterns in openwork.

Preserved in The Palace Museum

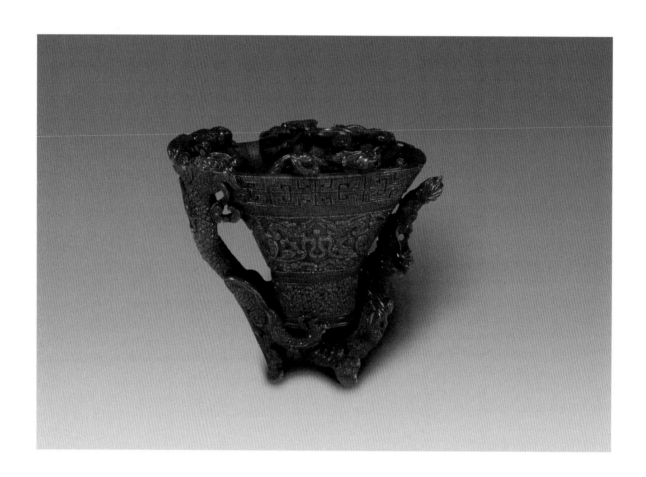

犀角雕龙柄螭龙纹杯

明末

犀角质

口径 8.5 ~ 13.5 厘米，足径 5 厘米，高 11.5 厘米

Rhinoceros Horn Cup with Carved Dragon Shaped Handle and Design

Late Ming Dynasty

Rhinoceros Horn

Mouth Diameter 8.5-13.5 cm/ Foot Diameter 5 cm/ Height 11.5 cm

敞口，上阔下窄，仿古觚形，以镂刻、浮雕技法，
将龙身作为杯柄与底足。龙身在右，龙尾在左，
头与上肢攀附在杯口，苍鳞、火焰布满全身。另
高浮雕三条小蛟龙，一条盘在大龙尾部，两条游
浮在杯口内侧，意为苍龙教子。杯壁自上而下装
饰方夔纹、双龙戏珠纹及浪花纹。

故宫博物院藏

The cup which resembles the ancient gu-vessel
has a flared mouth, a wide upper part and a narrow
lower part. The dragon's body is used as its
handle and foot. They are carved with the skills of
openwork and relief. The dragon's body is on the
right and the dragon's tail on the left with its head
and forelegs resting on the cup mouth. The dragon
is covered with carved dark green scales and
blazes. Three little flood dragons are engraved in
high relief: one is wreathing around the tail of the
big dragon, and the other two are swimming inside
the mouth of the cup, which has the meaning of "the
dragon's instructing its youngsters". The exterior
of the cup is decorated, from the top to the bottom,
with kui patterns, patterns of two dragons playing a
ball and spoondrift patterns.

Preserved in The Palace Museum

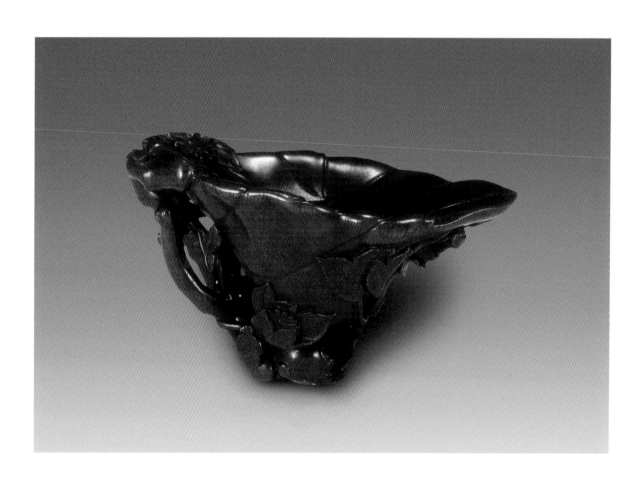

犀角雕芙蓉秋虫杯

明末

犀角质

口径 8.8 ~ 16 厘米，足径 3 ~ 4.4 厘米，高 9.2 厘米

Rhinoceros Horn Cup Carved with Hibiscus and Grasshopper

Late Ming Dynasty

Rhinoceros Horn

Mouth Diameter 8.8–16 cm / Foot Diameter 3–4.4 cm / Height 9.2 cm

亚洲犀牛角制。采用圆雕、镂刻技法，以芙蓉叶为杯，枝茎、花蕾为柄、足，杯壁四周又以野菊为衬，一只大腹蝈蝈低伏在叶片之上，津津有味地食着叶片。敞口的叶形杯底，呈沟壑状，筋脉隐显。此杯造型敦厚，刀法娴熟流畅，浑厚中见精雅。

故宫博物院藏

The cup is made of Asian rhinoceros horns. The cup, carved in openwork and circular engraving, is made into the shape of a hibiscus leaf, and uses the stems and buds of the flowers as its handle and foot. All around the cup wall are wild chrysanthemums. A big-belly grasshopper stoops over the flower leaf, chewing the leaves with relish. The leaf-shaped cup has a wide flared mouth. The ways of carving is elegant and exquisite and the design is magnificent and impressive.

Preserved in The Palace Museum

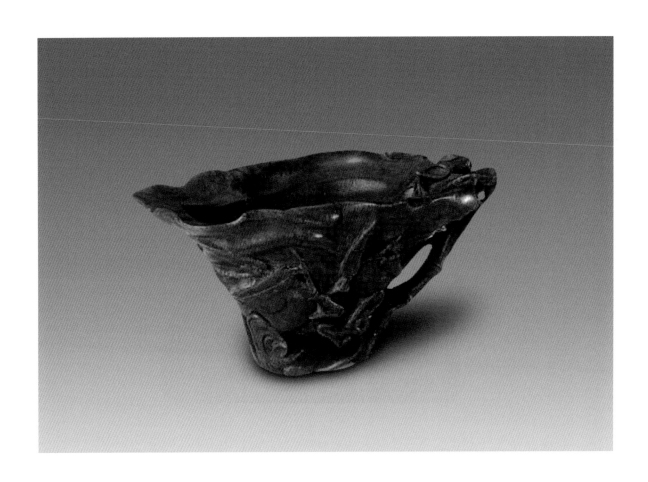

犀角雕竹子灵芝杯

明末

犀角质

口径 10.3 ～ 16.4 厘米，足径 3.3 ～ 5.6 厘米，高 7.8 厘米

Rhinoceros Horn Cup Carved with Design of Bamboo and Ganoderma

Late Ming Dynasty

Rhinoceros Horn

Mouth Diameter 10.3-16.4 cm/ Foot Diameter 3.3-5.6 cm/ Height 7.8 cm

杯形如斗，呈剖空灵芝状，口沿自然卷曲。
杯身有弦纹，印痕似水波晕散。杯身下镂雕
竹枝及灵芝为底，而杯錾则雕成竹茎、藤蔓
的造型。外壁还浮雕竹叶、灵芝的形状。

故宫博物院藏

The cup is shaped as a bucket. The cup looks
like a hollowed ganoderma with a natural curly
rim. The body has bow string patterns and
the moulage is like ripples spreading out. The
bottom part is carved with bamboo branches
and ganoderma in openwork and the handle
is carved into bamboo stems entwining with
tendrils and vines. The exterior wall of the cup
is engraved with bamboo leaves and ganoderma
in relief.

Preserved in The Palace Museum

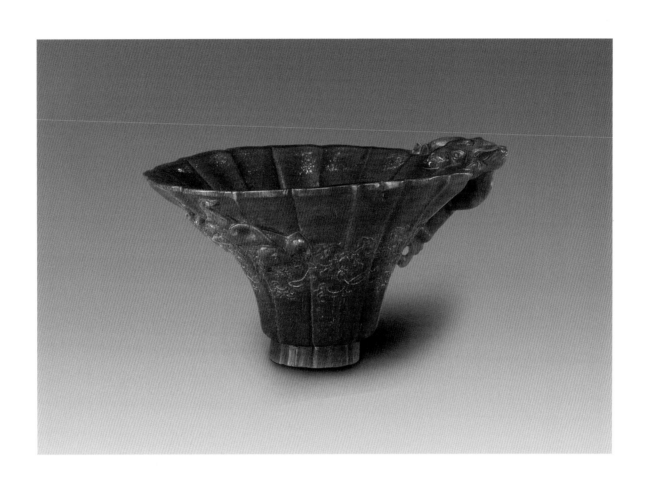

犀角雕螭纹菊瓣式杯

明末

犀角质

口径 10.3 ~ 14.3 厘米，足径 3.5 ~ 3.6 厘米，高 8 厘米

Rhinoceros Horn Cup Carved with Dragon Design and Chrysanthemum Petal

Late Ming Dynasty

Rhinoceros Horn

Mouth Diameter 10.3–14.3 cm/ Foot Diameter 3.5–3.6 cm/ Height 8 cm

通体雕成菊花初开式，敞口，敛腹，小底。杯口沿磨平，呈花瓣式，外壁浅浮雕缠枝宝相花纹，每一瓣上一朵。又高浮雕三螭攀爬，卷尾扭身，姿态各异，组成"S"形，打破了杯身花瓣式的垂直线条，与宝相花纹的环型构图也成对比，显示出高超的意匠。

故宫博物院藏

The entire cup is carved into the pattern of an early blossoming chrysanthemum. It has a flared mouth, a contracted belly and a little bottom. The rim of the mouth is ground and polished and is in the shape of a petal. The outer wall is a bas-relief of winding rosettes pattern, with one on each petal. Three dragons are carved in high relief in various postures, with their tails curled and bodies twisted into S shape. The design breaks the vertical lines of the petal-like body, and forms a comparison with the annular pattern of rosettes. The carving and the shape of the whole cup show an excellent and high level of craftman ideas.

Preserved in The Palace Museum

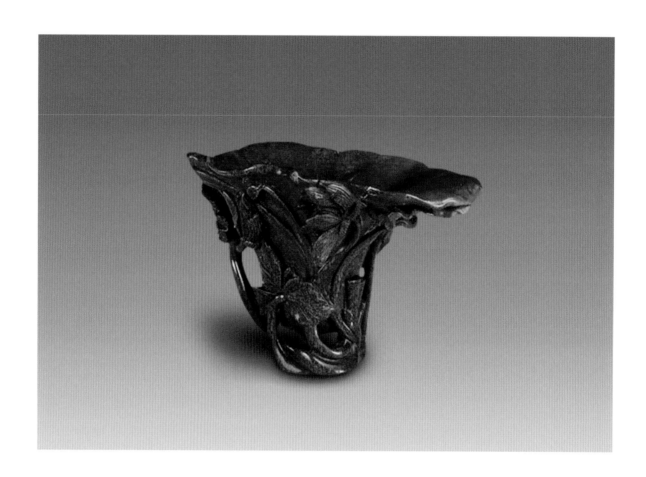

犀角雕荷花杯

明末

犀角质

口径 10.3 ~ 15.1 厘米，高 10.7 厘米

Rhinoceros Horn Cup Carved with Lotus Design

Late Ming Dynasty

Rhinoceros Horn

Mouth Diameter 10.3–15.1 cm/ Height 10.7 cm

杯身雕成一把莲式，主体为一大荷叶，卷曲
成筒，口沿敞开，外壁高浮雕荷叶、荷花，
杯下叶柄弯曲盘转成底足，造型舒放，荷花、
荷叶的形式均做了大胆夸张的手法处理。荷
叶的卷边、花瓣的开放都用高浮雕乃至圆雕
来表现，极富立体感。

故宫博物院藏

The cup is carved and shaped as a lotus. With
a broad mouth rim, the main part is a big
lotus leaf, crimping and curling like a drum.
The outer wall is engraved with lotus leaves
and blossoms in high relief. At the lower part
of the cup, leaf stalks curve and entwine to
form the bottom. The design is exquisite. The
shape of lotus leaves and blossoms are greatly
exaggerated. The curling rim of the leaves
and the blossomed petals are manifested in
high relief or even circular engraving, full of
stereoscopic sensation.

Preserved in The Palace Museum

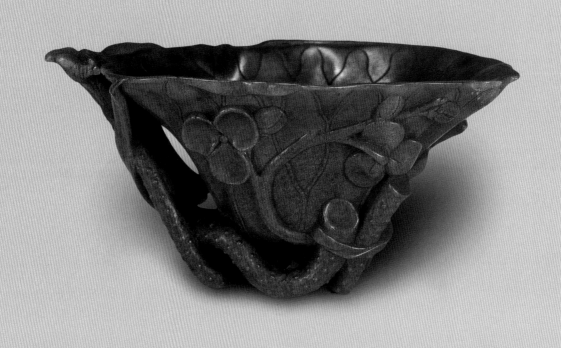

犀角雕莲蓬纹荷叶形杯

明末

犀角质

口径 10.2 ~ 17.2 厘米，高 8.5 厘米

荷叶上兜，侈口，呈盆状，三根叶茎茎刺突起交叉盘结于杯底，成为杯足。一茎连着叶杯，一茎端还残留有三片花瓣的莲蓬，一茎连着上卷如盒的小荷叶。杯壁有一束小海棠花。此件角杯除采用镂刻浮雕技法外，还使用了热烫衔接技法，使杯体之外的荷叶虬茎婉转，自然灵透。

故宫博物院藏

Rhinoceros Horn Cup Carved with Lotus Leaf Shape and Lotus Seedpod Pattern

Late Ming Dynasty

Rhinoceros Horn

Mouth Diameter 10.2-17.2 cm/ Height 8.5 cm

The cup looks like an upturned lotus leaf and its wide flared mouth is like a basin. Three leaf stalk thorns, which are protruding, crossing and winding at the bottom of the cup, form the foot of the cup. One stalk links with the handle; one stalk bears the remaining seedpods of the three petals and one links with an upwarping box-like little lotus leaf. The wall is incised with a bunch of begonias. The cup is carved in open work and relief as well as the skills of hot iron linking techniques, which fully display the natural, intricate and curly stalks of lotus leaves.

Preserved in The Palace Museum

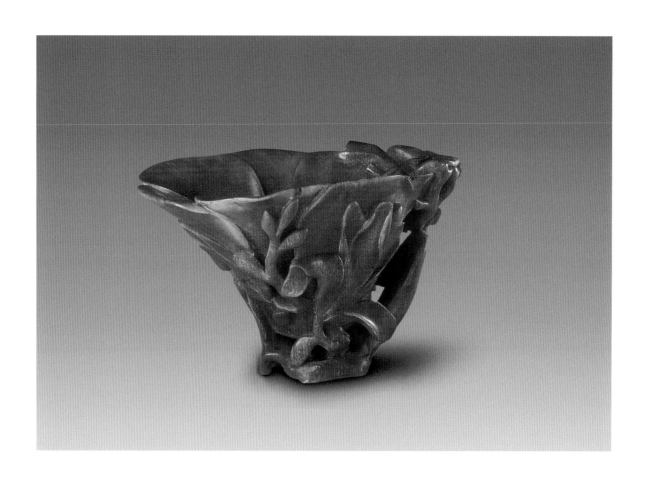

犀角镂雕玉兰花杯

明末

犀角质

口径 12.2 ～ 16.8 厘米，足径 7 ～ 7.8 厘米，高 8.1 厘米

Rhinoceros Horn Cup Carved with Magnolia Design

Late Ming Dynasty

Rhinoceros Horn

Mouth Diameter 12.2–16.8 cm/ Foot Diameter 7–7.8 cm/ Height 8.1 cm

棕红色，杯口呈椭圆形。匠人利用犀角上宽

下窄的自然形状，截取一段，并随形布势，

刻成玉兰花形，再在柄体上深浮雕枝、叶，

浅浮雕玉兰花瓣被花丛中的枝叶覆盖，使器

形整体看来，若花丛中的一朵大花。

故宫博物院藏

The brownish red cup has an oval-shaped mouth
rim. The sculptor, by employing the natural
shape of a rhinoceros horn which is broad at the
upper part and narrow at the bottom, cut one
part out of the horn and carved it into magnolia
flower according to its natural curves. The
handle is carved with branches and leaves in
deep relief and magnolia petals in bas-relief,
which is like a picture of flowers covered by
branches and leaves. The whole cup looks like a
big flower in anthemy.

Preserved in The Palace Museum

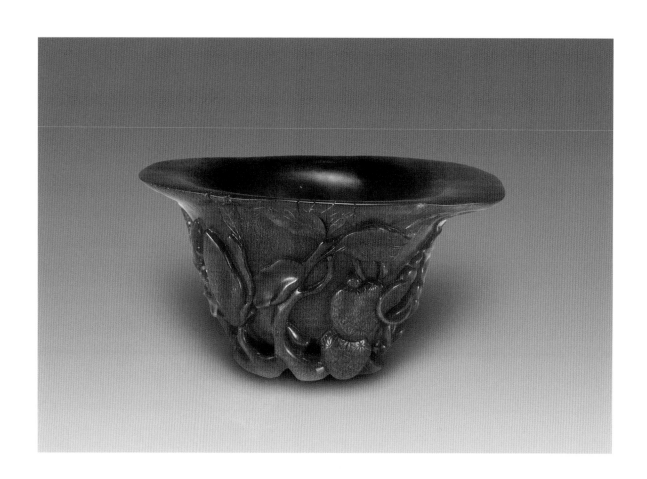

犀角雕玉兰花果杯

明末

犀角质

口径 12.2 ～ 16.8 厘米，足径 7 ～ 7.8 厘米，高 8.1 厘米

Rhinoceros Horn Cup Carved with Magnolia and Fruits Design

Late Ming Dynasty

Rhinoceros Horn

Mouth Diameter 12.2–16.8 cm/ Foot Diameter 7–7.8 cm/ Height 8.1 cm

该藏由亚洲大犀角雕刻而成。敞口，宽流，椭圆形，棕红色。杯身外壁浅浮雕葡萄、玉兰花、荔枝，花繁果茂，底足为镂刻盘枝。此杯大而不笨，浑朴中见精细，典雅中见豪放，是明代犀雕中之精品。

故宫博物院藏

The cup is made of Asian rhinoceros horn. The oval-shaped, brownish red cup has a flared mouth and a broad sprout. The outer wall of the cup is engraved with many flowers and fruits, including grapes, Yulan, and litchi in bas-relief. The bottom foot is carved with the design of tangled branches in open work. The cup is big but not cumbersome; simple, but with details. It is bold and elegant and was one of the masterpieces among the rhinoceros horn carvings in the Ming Dynasty.

Preserved in The Palace Museum

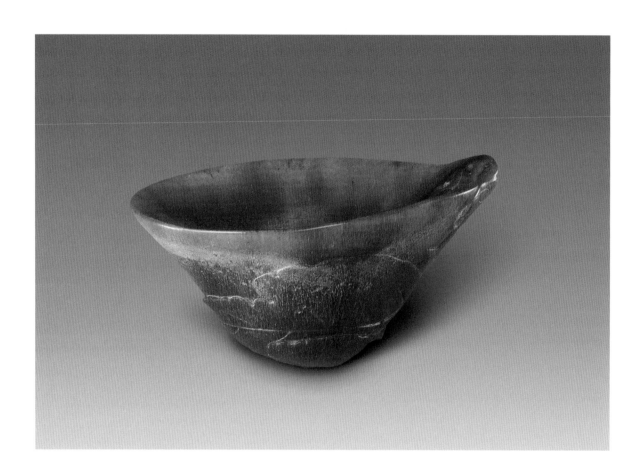

犀角雕双叶瓜形杯

明末

犀角质

口径 8.2 ～ 13.3 厘米，高 6 厘米

Rhinoceros Horn Cup Carved with Two Leaves and Melon Shape

Late Ming Dynasty

Rhinoceros Horn

Mouth Diameter 8.2-13.3 cm/ Height 6 cm

外壁浮雕连枝双叶，合抱杯身。匠人独具只眼，选择恰好符合犀角根部之形，只需翻转来用，略做处理，即成浅腹、敞口、曲线优美的杯体，其妙在似与不似之间。叶片的刻画尤见功力，翻卷、虫蚀等细节生动自然，廖廖几刀，添无穷意趣。杯口内的一片小叶，更成为点睛之笔。

故宫博物院藏

The outer wall of the cup is carved in relief with two leaves and branches which embrace the body of the cup. The sculptor, with a unique eye, chose the daily image which just fits the shape of the root of a rhinoceros horn. Simply turn the bottom and modify the appearance a little bit and it's easy to transform the horn into a cup with a shallow belly, a flared mouth and beautiful curves. The leaves are carved skillfully with vivid details of rolled worm-eaten parts. Interest and charm are displayed in a few carved lines. There is also a little leaf in the mouth which is undoubtedly the best part of the cup.

Preserved in The Palace Museum

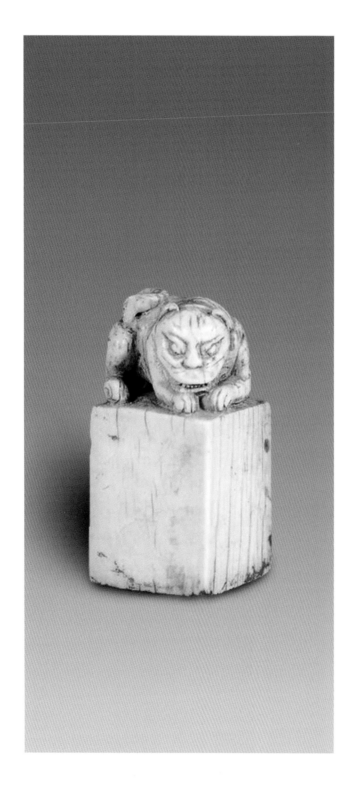

"仉砚香诊"象牙印

明

象牙质

宽 3 厘米，高 6 厘米

Ivory Seal

Ming Dynasty

Ivory

Width 3 cm/ Height 6 cm

印钮为虎形，呈静蹲状。此印是仉砚香医生
处方用印。

上海中医药博物馆藏

The collection was a private seal of a doctor
whose name was Zhang Yanxiang. The knob of
the seal is in the shape of a quiet squatting tiger.
When the doctor made prescriptions for his
patients, he stamped the seal instead of writing
his name on the prescriptions.

Preserved in Shanghai Museum of Traditional
Chinese Medicine

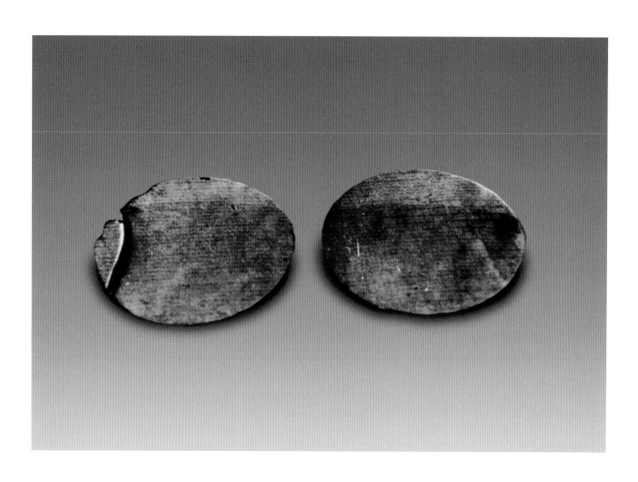

眼镜镜片

明

水晶质

直径 4.1 厘米，厚 0.15 厘米

Spectacle Lens

Ming Dynasty

Crystal

Diameter 4.1 cm/ Thickness 0.15 cm

此镜为凸透镜。出土时尚见金属镜架，因朽
坏未能保存。1972 年乐山长征制药厂工地明
墓出土。

乐山大佛乌尤文物保护管理局藏

The eyeglasses are convex lens. The metal glass
frames and legs were still available when the
glasses were discovered. It failed to be kept
because it was rusting and damaged. They were
unearthed in a Ming tomb at the construction
site of Changzheng Pharmaceutical Factory,
Leshan City, Sichuan Province, in 1972.
Preserved in Leshan Giant Buddha Cultural
relics protection administration of Wuyou

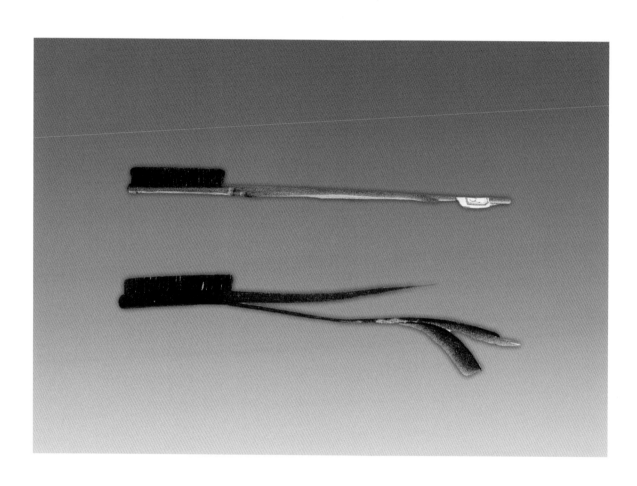

猪鬃穿牛角柄药刷

明

犀角质

长 14.8 厘米

Medicine Brush with Bristles Threading into Ox Horn

Ming Dynasty

Rhinoceros Horn

Length 14.8 cm

用作制药辅助工具。江苏省江阴市夏颧墓
出土。

江阴博物馆藏

The brushes were utilized as an auxiliary tool
for making medicine and were unearthed
in Xiaquan's tomb, Jiangyin City, Jiangsu
Province.

Preserved in Jiangyin Museum

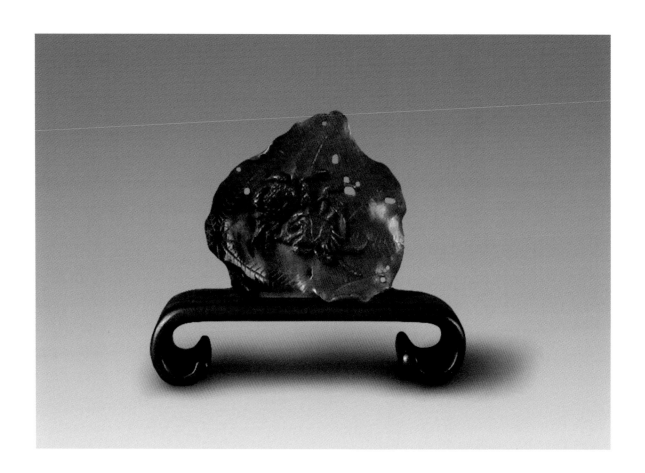

犀角荷叶蟹雕

明

犀角质

宽 6.4 厘米，高 7.6 厘米

Rhinoceros Horn Carving with Design of Crab on Lotus Leaf

Ming Dynasty

Rhinoceros Horn

Width 6.4 cm/ Height 7.6 cm

荷叶形，为犀角雕成荷叶状，上有双蟹浮雕，雕工细腻，磨制光滑。工艺品，具较高观赏及收藏价值。1959 年入藏，保存完好。

中华医学会 / 上海中医药大学医史博物馆藏

The artware is in the shape of a lotus leaf. The rhinoceros horn is carved into a lotus leaf on which are two crabs engraved in relief. With fine and smooth craftsmanship and smoothly polishing, it has high appreciation and collection value. It was collected in 1959 and is still in good condition.

Preserved in Chinese Medical Association/ Museum of Chinese Medicine, Shanghai University of Traditional Chinese Medicine

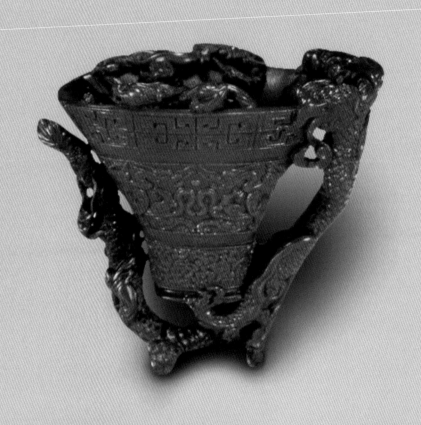

犀角雕龙柄螭龙纹杯

明

犀角质

口长径 13.5 厘米，短径 8.5 厘米，足径 5 厘米，高 11.5 厘米

杯口外撇，上阔下窄，仿古觚形。图形有"苍龙教子"之意。

1985 年，香港著名医生、医学博士、文物收藏家叶义捐献。

故宫博物院藏

Rhinoceros Horn Cup with Carved Dragon Shaped Handle and Design

Ming Dynasty

Rhinoceros Horn

Major Mouth Diameter 13.5 cm/ Minor Mouth Diameter 8.5 cm/ Foot Diameter 5 cm/ Height 11.5 cm

The cup which resembles the ancient gu-vessel has a flared mouth, a wide upper part and a narrow lower part. Motifs decorating on the body have the meaning of "the black dragon's instructing its youngsters". It was donated by Ye Yi, one of the famous Hong Kong doctors, Doctor of Medicine and cultural relic collector, in 1985.

Preserved in The Palace Museum

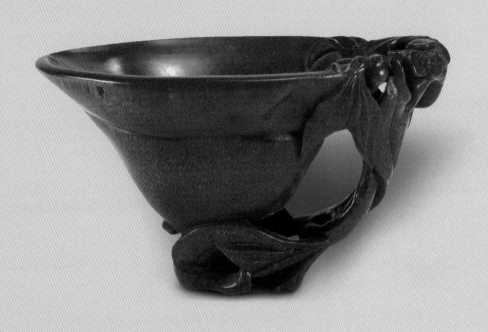

犀角桃式杯

明

犀角质

口长径 14.3 厘米，短径 9.2 厘米，高 8.8 厘米

杯体随形，敞口呈桃式，底收小，镂雕桃枝及果，

叶作杯柄，延至杯底成为底座。

故宫博物院藏

Rhinoceros Horn Cup Carved with Peach Shape Design

Ming Dynasty

Rhinoceros horn

Major Mouth Diameter 14.3cm/ Minor Mouth Diameter 9.2 cm/ Height 8.8 cm

The cup uses the natural form of the rhinoceros horn. It has a peach-shaped flared mouth and a contracted bottom. It is engraved with the design of peach tree branches and fruits in open work. The handle is in the shape of a peach leaf which extends to the cup bottom and forms the pedestal of the cup.

Preserved in The Palace Museum

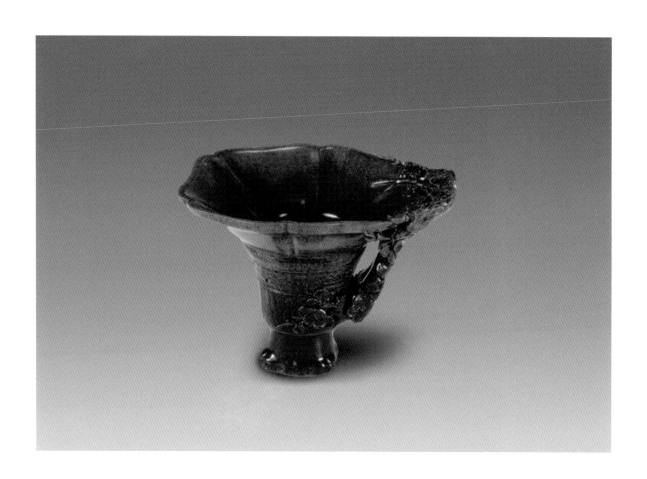

犀角杯

明

犀角质

口径 16.2 厘米，高 12.3 厘米

Rhinoceros Horn Cup

Ming Dynasty

Rhinoceros Horn

Mouth Diameter 16.2 cm/ Height 12.3 cm

依犀角原状雕刻成形。喇叭口外敞，口下急收成浅圆腹，四方委角花瓣式圈足，外壁一侧有枝梅形柄，上端的梅花与杯口相接，下端梅花至杯腹。腹上部饰夔纹一周，下饰蕉叶纹一周。口沿和足边各雕回纹一周。

河北博物院藏

The cup uses the natural form of the rhinoceros horn. It has a trumpet-like flared mouth, a contracted shallow round belly, and a ring foot with petals on the corners. The handle on the exterior wall is shaped as a plum tree. The plum blossom on the upper part connects with the mouth while the one on the lower part extends to the cup belly. A circle of Kui pattern is decorated around the upper body and a circle of banana leaf pattern is carved around the lower part. A pattern which looks like the Chinese character "Hui" is carved respectively around the rim of the mouth and the edge of the ring foot.

Preserved in Hebei Museum

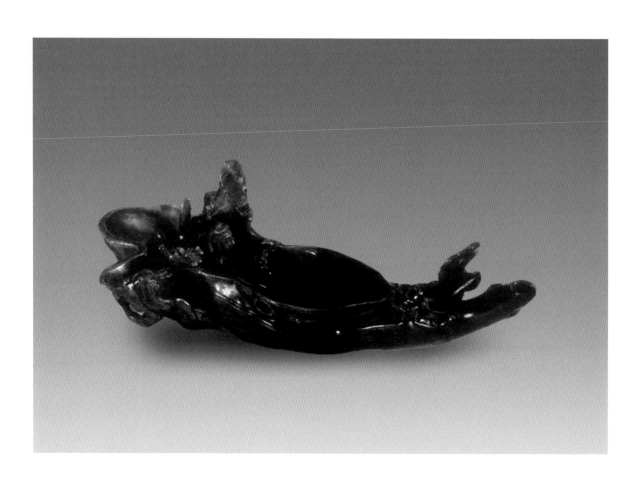

仙人乘槎犀角杯

明

犀角质

长 26.5 厘米，高 8.6 厘米，重 261.5 克

Rhinoceros Horn Cup Carved with Immortal Design

Ming Dynasty

Rhinoceros Horn

Length 26.5 cm/ Height 8.6 cm/ Weight 261.5 g

雕刻艺人选用一支上乘的犀角，以仙人乘槎凌空到达天河的神话故事为题材，依犀角的自然形状，雕刻成树槎形一叶扁舟。以角根为槎尾，以角梢为槎头，角梢处有一圆形充满孔，槎身和槎底环绕浮雕的流水纹，槎内端坐着一位老者靠假山和枯木。艺人采用圆雕、透雕、浮雕和浅刻相结合的技法，使整个作品层次丰富，雕刻精湛。它既是一件极佳的工艺品，又是一种清凉、解毒的实用酒具，且具有很高的经济价值。1961 年扬州市福利公司捐赠。

扬州博物馆藏

Using the natural form and high quality of a rhinoceros horn, the sculptor carved it into a tiny tree-like raft. The moral of the sculpture was based on a fairy story that an immortal was flying high in the air to the Milky Way by a raft. The root part is made into the stern of the raft and the sharp is made into the bow. There is a round hole at the sharp of the horn. The body and the bottom of the raft are carved with patterns of running water. On the raft, an old man is resting against a withered tree and a rockery. The sculptor combined the skills of circular engravure, openwork, relief and intaglio to make the work well-arranged. The ware is an exquisite carving craft. It is not only an excellent artware, but also a practical wine vessel which has the function of cooling blood, reducing heat and detoxifying. The item has high economic value and was donated by Benefits Company, Yangzhou City, in 1961.

Preserved in Yangzhou Museum

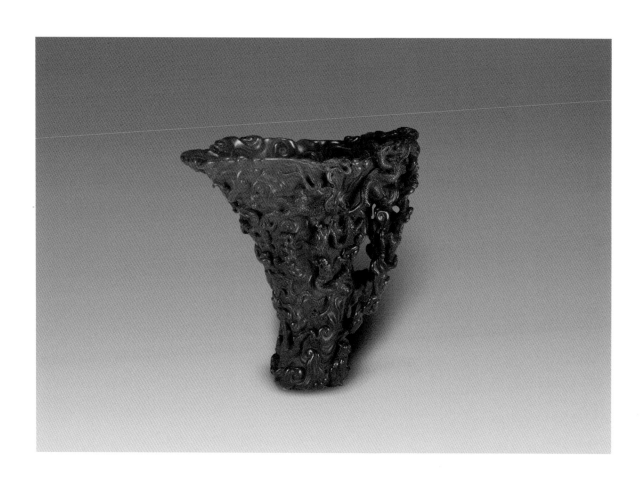

犀角雕云龙杯

明末清初

犀角质

口径 11.5 ~ 19.5 厘米，底径 7.3 厘米，高 21.3 厘米

Rhinoceros Horn Cup Carved with Dragons in Clouds

Late Ming Dynasty/ Early Qing Dynasty

Rhinoceros Horn

Mouth Diameter11.5 -19.5 cm/ Foot Diameter 7.3 cm/ Height 21.3 cm

栗色。呈宽流爵杯形，随犀角自然形状雕刻而成，镂花天然形双股式把，下为圆柱形，平底。通体以高浮雕技法雕云纹，云中隐现九龙，或飞于杯口，或盘绕于双把，或腾跃凌空相戏，气势壮观。此杯是明代犀角雕刻工艺中的珍品。

故宫博物院藏

The chestnut cup uses the natural form of the rhinoceros horn and is carved into the shape of Jue (an ancient wine vessel with three legs) with a broad spout. The ornamental engraving with double-strand handle is in openwork. It has a cylindrical lower part and a flat bottom. Its exterior is carved, in high relief, with cloud patterns. Nine dragons are in the clouds: some rest on the mouth and handle; some fly in the clouds. With dragons and clouds, the design is magnificent and impressive. It was a treasure among the rhinoceros horn carvings in the Ming Dynasty.

Preserved in The Palace Museum

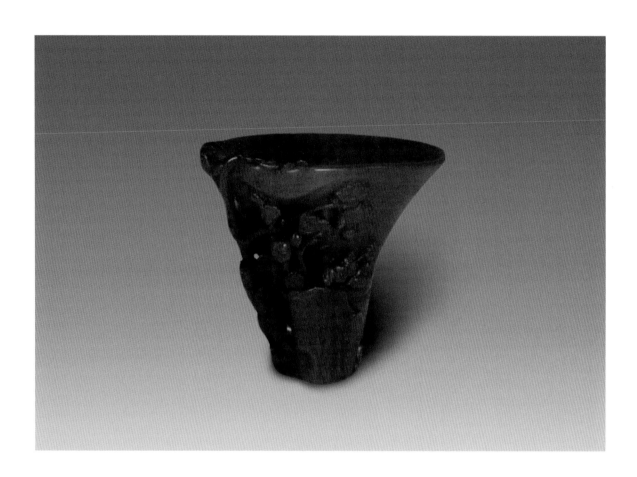

尤侃犀角雕芙蓉鸳鸯杯

明末清初

犀角质

口径 8 ~ 12 厘米，足径 3 ~ 4.5 厘米，高 8.3 厘米

Rhinoceros Horn Cup with Designs of Hibiscus and Mandarin Ducks by You Kan

Late Ming Dynasty/Early Qing Dynasty

Rhinoceros Horn

Mouth Diameter 8–12 cm / Foot Diameter 3–4.5 cm / Height 8.3 cm

侈口，束足，平底形杯。杯柄由山石花枝组成，花枝上挺，直延入杯口之内。花枝右侧以山石为主，左侧浅浮刻溪河，一对鸳鸯相伴栖于花茎之下。在杯底刻有阴文"直生""尤侃"篆体方圆印各一个。

故宫博物院藏

The cup has a wide flared mouth, a contracted foot and a flat bottom. The handle consists of the patterns of carved hills, rocks and hibiscus flowers which extend upward into the rim of the cup. Rocks and stones are mainly on the right of the flowers while on the left of the flowers it is incised with a river in relief. A pair of mandarin ducks is perching under the flowers. There are two seals incised in intaglio at the bottom of the cup; one is square and the other is round. The two seals are incised in seal scripts (Zhuan style) with the Chinese characters reading "Zhisheng" and "Youkan".
Preserved in The Palace Museum

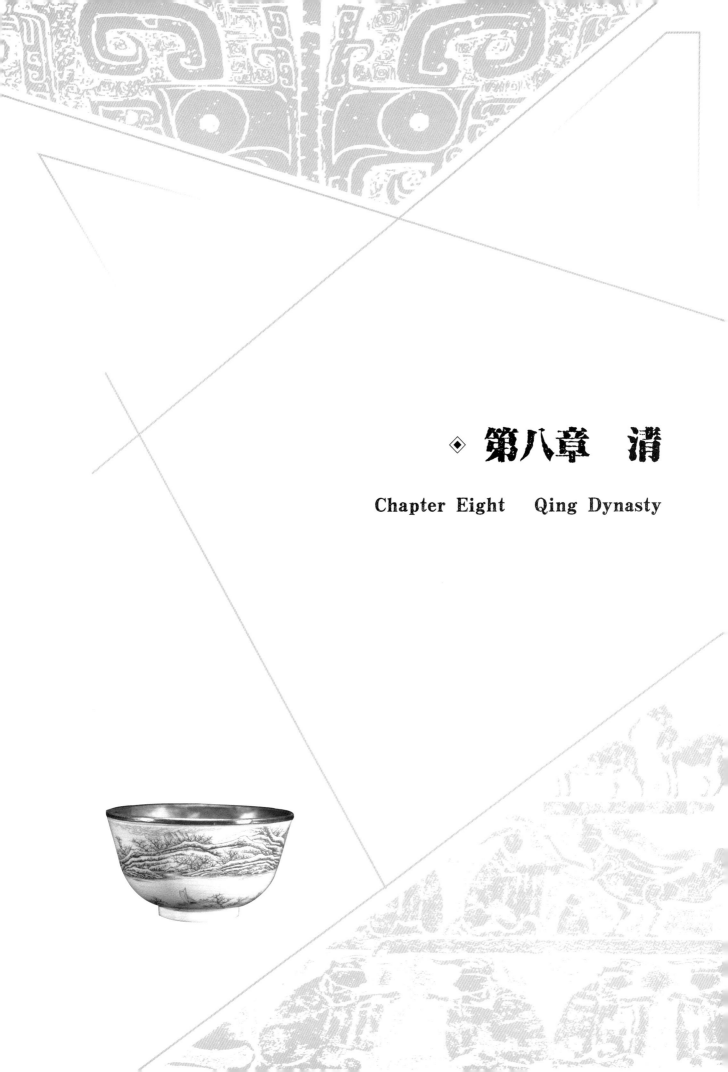

◆ 第八章　清

Chapter Eight　Qing Dynasty

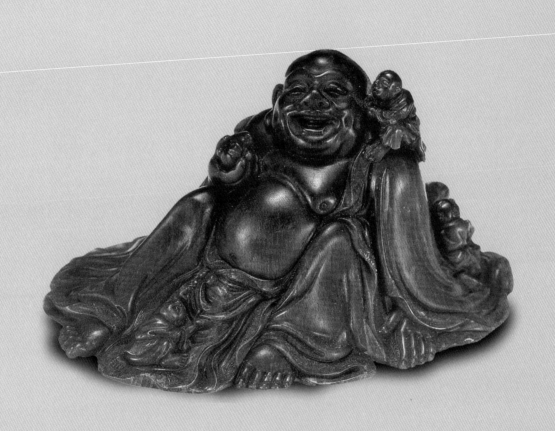

犀角雕弥勒佛

清初

犀角质

底径 5.3 ～ 10 厘米，高 7.9 厘米

用亚洲犀牛额前的小角雕刻而成。上深下浅，呈蒸栗色，底凹洼处填有木片以保护其微薄的雕刻边角。弥勒广袖长衣，赤足曲肱，仰首倚袋而坐。他的身前、背后有四个小童，有的给他抻衣，有的给他掏耳挠痒。弥勒缩颈耸肩，张口大笑。此物是清代初期犀角雕刻中的趣味之作。

故宫博物院藏

Rhinoceros Horn Statue Carved with Maitreya Buddha

Early Qing Dynasty

Rhinoceros Horn

Bottom Diameter 5.3–10 cm/ Height 7.9 cm

The Maitreya Buddha is made of the small horn on the forehead of Asian rhinoceros. The ware is chestnut which is dark at the upper part and light at the lower part of the statuette. Some wood chips are stuffed in the concave part of the statue in order to protect the corners and edges of the delicate sculpture. With his arms bent behind, resting against a bag and sitting with his chin up, the Buddha is bare-footed and wears a long robe with wide sleeves. Four little boys are around him, some helping to stretch his clothes, some scratching itches for him. The Buddha is so pleased that he laughs happily with his neck and shoulder contracted and shrugged and mouth open. This artistic work of rhinoceros horn was full of fun and interests in the early Qing Dynasty.

Preserved in The Palace Museum

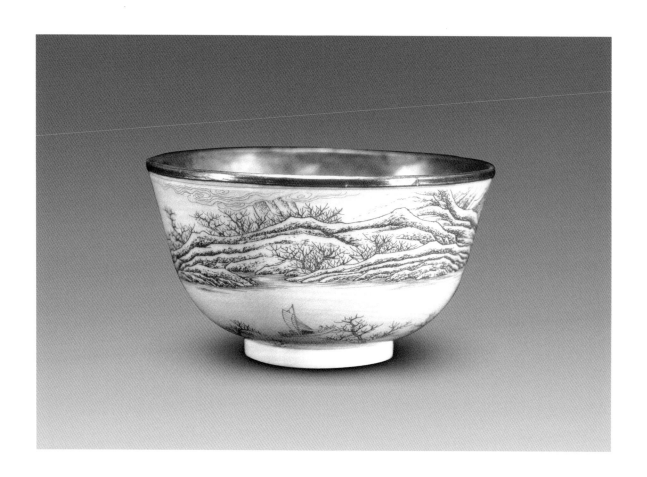

象牙雕山水银里碗

清初

象牙质

口径 9.2 厘米，底径 4.3 厘米，高 5.3 厘米

Ivory Bowl with Silver Lining and Carved with Landscape Designs

Early Qing Dynasty

Ivory

Mouth Diameter 9.2 cm/ Bottom Diameter 4.3 cm/ Height 5.3 cm

圆形，敞口，圈足，"宫制"篆文款。该藏是宫中喝奶茶之用具。碗内镶有银里。匠人以浅刻、填色等技法，在碗壁上刻峰岭起伏，峭壁如嶂，岩壁之下，江面微波荡漾。一叶小舟顺流行驶，舟中一人在船头低首下视，一人在后抄桨掌舵。山中云雾缭绕，矮树丛生，枝秃叶落，一群鸿雁排成人字望空而行。并刻五言诗"来雁清霜后，孤帆远树中"，表达了作者的思乡之情。

故宫博物院藏

The round bowl has a flared mouth and a ring foot. The bowl was for drinking milky tea in the palace. It is inscribed with seal characters reading "Gong Zhi" (Made for the palace). The interior of the bowl is inlaid with silver lining. The exterior of the bowl is carved with rolling hills and steep cliffs through shallow carving and color-filling, under which is a rippling river. In the design, a little boat is floating down the river, and one man standing on the boat is lowering his head watching the river; the other man standing at the stern is paddling and steering the boat. Clouds and mists embrace the mountains where the thick shrubs have bare branches because their leaves are already fallen, and a flock of swan geese herringboned are flying in the sky. A poem with five characters is inscribed on it, which expresses the poet's homesickness.

Preserved in The Palace Museum

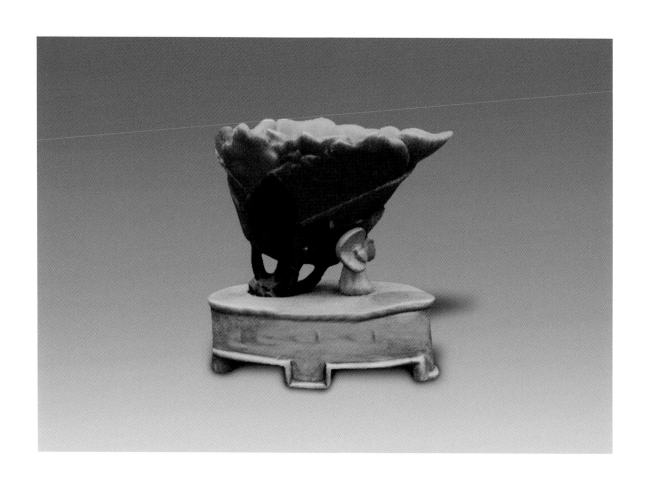

莲花犀角杯

清初

犀角质

口长径 6.6 厘米，口短径 4.25 厘米，通高 8 厘米，重 21 克

Rhinoceros Horn Cup Carved with Lotus Designs

Early Qing Dynasty

Rhinoceros Horn

Mouth Long Diameter 6.6 cm/ Mouth Short 4.25 cm/ Height 8 cm/ Weight 21 g

此为犀角制的艺术品，杯口呈莲花瓣状，用于装

饰。犀角，犀科动物犀牛的角，可作中药。

广东中医药博物馆藏

The rim of the cup is in the shape of a lotus petal.
The cup was utilized for decoration. Rhinoceros
horn is the horn of a rhinocerotidae animal. It can be
utilized as traditional Chinese medicine.
Preserved in Guangzhou Chinese Medicine Museum

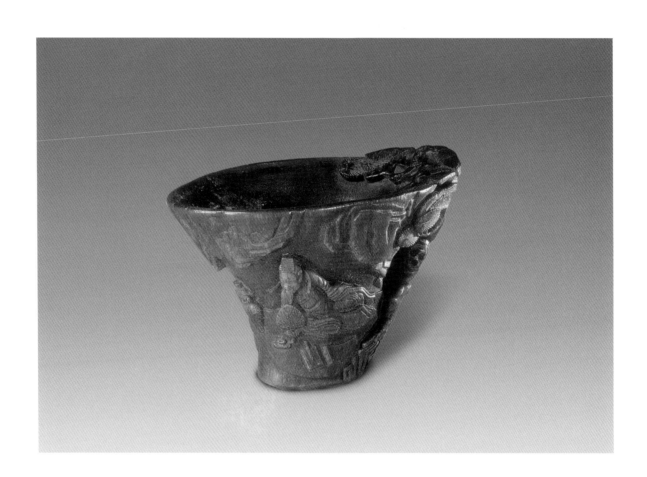

犀角雕太白醉酒杯

清初

犀角质

口径 9.3 ～ 14.1 厘米，底径 3.5 ～ 5 厘米，高 9 厘米

Rhinoceros Horn Cup Carved with Drunken Image of Li Po

Early Qing Dynasty

Rhinoceros Horn

Mouth Diameter 9.3-14.1 cm/ Bottom Diameter 3.5-5 cm/ Height 9 cm

随形、敞口，作品以透空镂雕技法，在犀角的一侧刻一古松为柄，松干苍鳞密结。又以浮雕技法，将古松顶枝上弯，横斜天矫，形若虬龙攀在杯口之内。崖下平台之上太白头戴乌纱幞头，身着长衣，髯须垂胸，左手抚膝，右手撑扇，盘膝曲肱，斜身侧卧闭目做沉思状。在他头前有两个酒坛，他的身前置有一杯、一碟、一砚、一笔和一张展开的纸卷。杯底刻有阴文"方宏斋制"篆体长方印。

故宫博物院藏

The cup uses the natural form of the rhinoceros horn. The cup has an elliptical open mouth and is carved in openwork. An aged-pine tree with thick dark green trunk is engraved as the handle on one side of the cup. The top branches of the pine, carved upward in oblique and exquisite curves with the relief carving skills, look like a qiu-dragon climbing on the rim. On the platform under the cliff, Li Po, who wears a black gauze cap and a long coat, and with his beard drooping to his chest, is stroking his knees with his left hand, and holding a fan in his right hand. Crossing his legs and bending his arms, Li Po, in the appearance of deep thinking, is lying on his side with his eyes closed. There are two wine jars beside his head. A cup, a dish, an ink stone, a brush and an unfolded paper are in front of him. The bottom of the cup is engraved with a rectangular marking with the seal characters in intaglio "Fang Hongzhai Zhi" (Made by Fanghongzhai).

Preserved in The Palace Museum

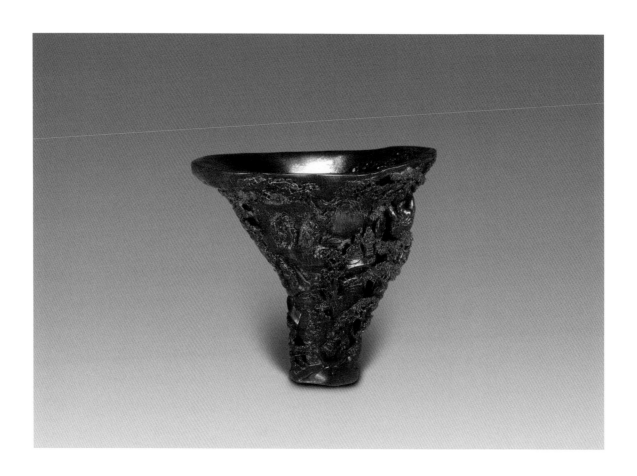

犀角雕山水人物杯

清初

犀角质

口径 10.2 ~ 15.8 厘米，足径 4.3 ~ 4.8 厘米，高 13.9 厘米

Rhinoceros Horn Cup Carved with Landscape and Figures Designs

Early Qing Dynasty

Rhinoceros Horn

Mouth Diameter 10.2-15.8 cm/ Foot Diameter 4.3-4.8 cm/ Height 13.9 cm

亚洲犀角制。棕色。磨口，切底，采用镂刻高浮雕技法，

以《西园雅集》中的《文聚图》为题材，制成敞口缩

足的觚形杯。杯身镂雕双树为柄，山景为衬，奇松、

古柏、枫、桐满植其间，山间溪流蜿蜒，小桥凌空平架，

十六个人物分为八组，或坐卧饮酒，或站立相迎送，

或聚合聊谈，吟诗论画，奋笔疾书。结构严谨，层次

分明。

故宫博物院藏

The brown cup is made of Asian rhinoceros horn. The rim of the cup is grinded and the bottom is cut. The cup is made according to the painting of *Wen Ju Painting* in *Hsi Yuan Ya Chi* with the techniques of openwork carving in high relief. It is in the shape of a drinking vessel and has a flared mouth and narrow foot. The cup is engraved with two trees as a handle. Mountains are the background where grow strangely-shaped pines, antique cypresses, maples, and sycamores. A small bridge crosses a creeping gurgling brook. The sixteen figures in eight groups carved on the body are either sitting or lying there drinking, or standing there welcoming or seeing-off friends, or chatting together, reciting poems, commenting on the paintings or writing swiftly respectively. The whole pattern is rigorous and coherent.

Preserved in The Palace Museum

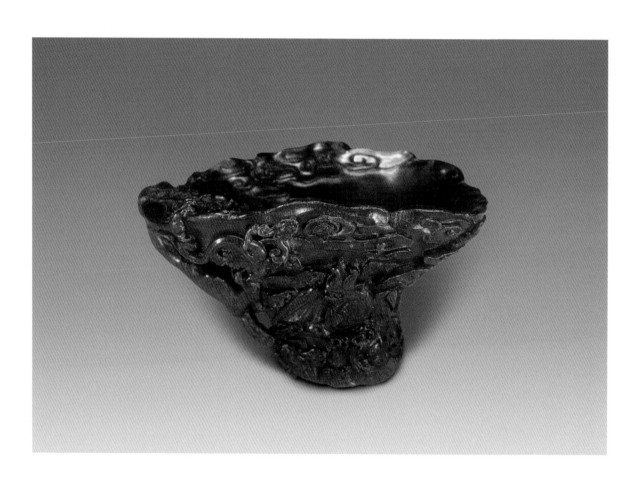

犀角雕水兽纹杯

清初

犀角质

口径 10.8 ~ 16.2 厘米，足径 4.7 ~ 5 厘米，高 9.5 厘米

Rhinoceros Horn Cup Carved with Water Beasts Design

Early Qing Dynasty

Rhinoceros Horn

Mouth Diameter 10.8-16.2 cm/ Foot Diameter 4.7-5 cm/ Height 9.5 cm

亚洲犀角制。粗短纯厚，上宽下窄。染色，色如蒸栗。采用深浮雕技法，在杯体外侧满刻各种水族异兽，有龟、螭、龙、夔、麒麟、牛、蟾、螺贝等。一条苍龙双臂紧攀杯口，龙身为杯柄，龙首窥伸入杯口之内，似在偷饮琼浆玉液。此杯雕刻图案繁密，刀技精湛，气势雄浑，是清代初期江苏一带高手制作。

故宫博物院藏

The cup is made of Asian rhinoceros horn. It is thick and short in form, broad on the top and narrow at the bottom. The cup is dyed in the color of steamed chestnut. The exterior of the cup is decorated with various carved water beasts in high relief such as turtles, chi-dragons, dragons, kui beasts, kylins, oxes, toads and shellfish. A black dragon is grasping the cup tightly with its two forearms; the body part of the dragon is made into the handle and the dragon head is peeping into the cup as if to sip the precious beverage surreptitiously. Dense in patterns, exquisite in techniques, and powerful in momentum, this cup was made by a master-hand from the area of Jiangsu Province in the early Qing Dynasty.

Preserved in The Palace Museum

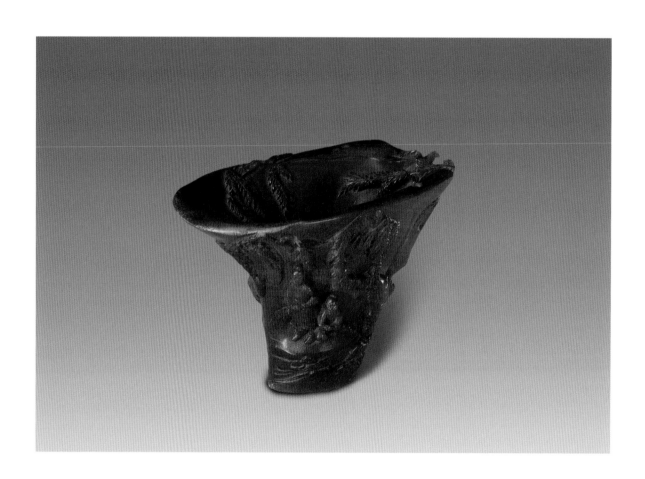

犀角雕柳荫牧马图杯

清初

犀角质

口径 9.5 ～ 14.6 厘米，足径 3.6 ～ 4.8 厘米，高 9.7 厘米

Rhinoceros Horn Cup Carved with Drawing of Raising Horse under Willow Trees

Early Qing Dynasty

Rhinoceros horn

Mouth Diameter 9.5-14.6 cm/ Foot Diameter 3.6-4.8 cm/ Height 9.7 cm

杯敞口，敛底，外壁浮雕两人于溪岸上，一立一坐，立者手执柳条，坐者手挽衣袖，目光所聚，为一健马，欢然翻滚于草丛之中，情景历历如在眼前。又雕岩石林立，形成杯耳，树枝轻扬，直入杯口内。下有溪水潺湲，流转如丝。此杯高浮雕技法十分纯熟，风格亦清新明快，并为同类题材犀角雕中所仅见，更显珍贵。

故宫博物院藏

The cup has a flared mouth and a contracted bottom. Two men carved on the exterior surface are standing or sitting on a creek bank. The standing man is holding a willow branch while the sitting man is rolling up his sleeves. Both are gazing at a strong horse which is joyfully rolling over in the grass. The scene is so vivid and it seems that it is visible before the eyes. The carved rocks form the cup handle and the slight swinging branches extend into the cup. The creek is flowing slowly like silk. With practiced high relief skills, the style is fresh and bright, which is the only artware of its kind in the rhinoceros horn carvings and becomes even more precious.

Preserved in The Palace Museum

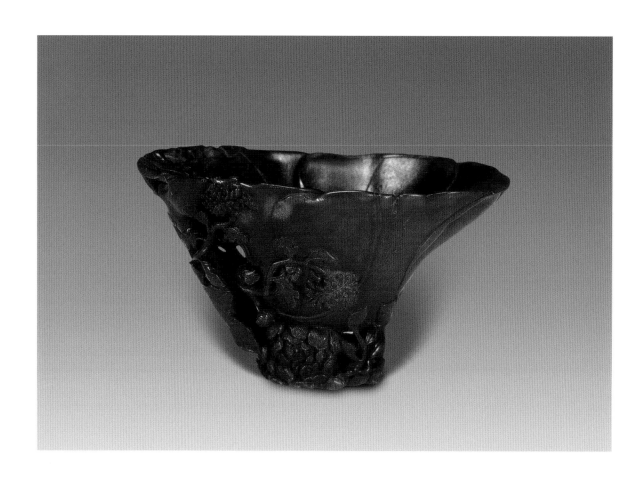

犀角雕花鸟杯

清初

犀角质

口径 10.4 ~ 15.6 厘米，足径 4.1 ~ 5.1 厘米，高 9 厘米

Rhinoceros Horn Cup Carved with Birds and Flowers

Early Qing Dynasty

Rhinoceros Horn

Mouth Diameter 10.4-15.6 cm/ Foot Diameter 4.1-5.1 cm/ Height 9 cm

亚洲犀牛角刻制。敞口，缩足，棕红色。杯身以芙蓉花为形，花瓣连体上兜，如半开状。盛开的花和茎叶盘结为底足。枝干为柄。还有两支妖娆的寿菊依着杯外壁而生。在杯内，一支带蕾花枝伸入杯底，两只小燕相随，枝上枝下跳跃嬉戏。

故宫博物院藏

The brownish red cup is made of the Asian rhinoceros horn, with a wide opening and a contracted ring foot. The body is in the shape of a hibiscus and the petals connect the top section and in the form of a half-blooming flower. The blooming flower and leaves entwine and form the foot of the cup while the branches become the handle. Two enchanting marigolds grow against the exterior wall of the cup. Inside the cup, a branch of buds extends to the bottom with two little swallows jumping up and down on the branches.

Preserved in The Palace Museum

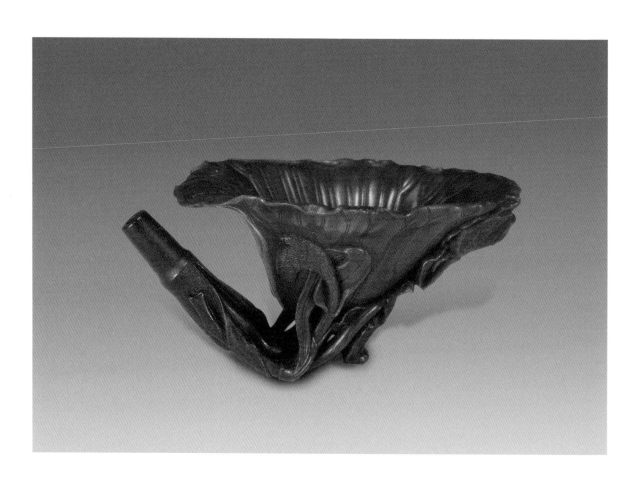

犀角雕莲蓬荷叶形杯

清初

犀角质

口径 10.6 ～ 16.8 厘米，高 16 厘米

Rhinoceros Horn Cup Carved with Lotus Leaves

Early Qing Dynasty

Rhinoceros Horn

Mouth Diameter 10.6-16.8 cm/ Height 16 cm

广角制。为流口内弯上翘、杯口敞阔外撇的荷叶形状。叶杯筋脉根根遒劲，杯下镂刻荷花，花心结有莲蓬，点衬的小荷叶微卷，与蒲草组成花枝，平展成底座，架住叶柄。杯内底有一洞与吸口相通，托住叶杯，不用倾斜，可将酒水吸入口中。

故宫博物院藏

The cup is made of rhinoceros horn. The craftsman carved the long horn into a lotus-shaped cup. The head part curves inward and is tip-tilted. The rim of the cup is open wide and flared. The ribs of the lotus root are vigorous and obvious. Enchased lotus flowers are blooming at the bottom. With flower pistil knotting the seedpod, lotus seeds are growing in the center. The small leaves, combining with leaf cattail and forming a branch, become the cup base and supporting the leaf handle. A hole at the bottom connects a suction port, through which wine can be sucked into mouth without tilting the cup.

Preserved in The Palace Museum

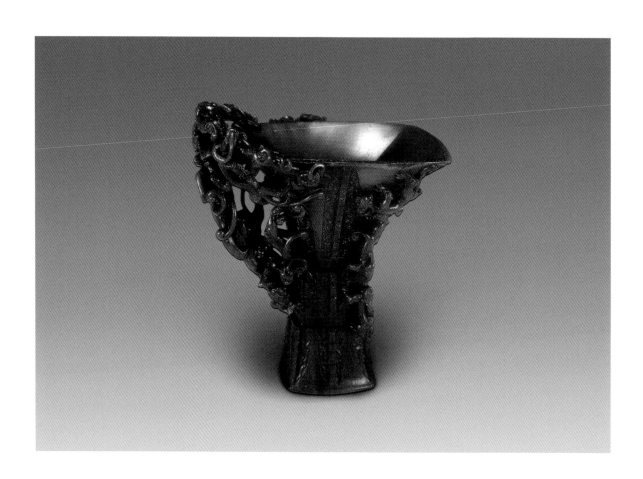

犀角雕螭纹杯

清中期

犀角质

口径 10 ~ 17.5 厘米，足径 3.1 ~ 4.2 厘米，高 16.2 厘米

Rhinoceros Horn Cup Carved with Dragon Designs

Mid-Qing Dynasty

Rhinoceros Horn

Mouth Diameter 10-17.5 cm/ Foot Diameter 3.1-4.2 cm/ Height 16.2 cm

杯身较长，腰细，底甚阔，口大而平，且有八棱，形如古觚。口下与足上雕饰古蕉叶纹，腹部雕饰雷纹为地，通体透雕和浮雕蟠螭15 只。

故宫博物院藏

The cup has a long body, a thin waist and a broad bottom. Its eight-edged mouth is big and flat. The cup is shaped as an ancient goblet. The part below the mouth and above the foot is carved with banana leaf pattern; the belly is carved with thunder lines. The whole cup is carved with 15 hydras in relief and openwork.

Preserved in The Palace Museum

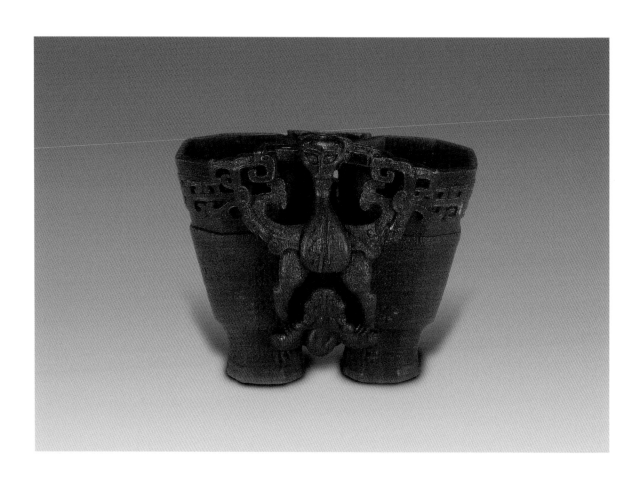

犀角雕英雄杯

清中期

犀角质

口径 5.6 ~ 15 厘米，足径 3.9 ~ 10.4 厘米，高 13.2 厘米

Rhinoceros Horn Cup Carved with Hero Image

Mid-Qing Dynasty

Rhinoceros Horn

Mouth Diameter 5.6-15 cm/ Foot Diameter 3.9-10.4 cm/ Height 13.2 cm

此器中间为双螭，左右各一杯，杯体高而方，形如古尊。有八棱。口沿雕回纹，通体雕兽面纹，双杯中间上下各有一只螭穿过，正面上方螭的双爪按在下方螭的双肩上，身子向后形成自然弯曲状，似成杯柄。反面的上方有一兽首，左右各有一只小螭相向而立。

故宫博物院藏

The connection part of the twin cups is carved with two chi-dragons. Each cup with octagonal edges is high and square in the shape of an ancient wine vessel. The mouth rim is carved with meandering patterns. The entire body of the cup is engraved with beast-face veins. The two Chi-dragons standing on the top and bottom of the cup respectively are interlacing. On the observe side, the upper Chi-dragon which bends backward naturally as the handle, is pressing its two claws on the shoulders of the one at the bottom. On the reverse side, a beast head is carved on the top with two little Chi-dragons standing face to face on each side.

Preserved in The Palace Museum

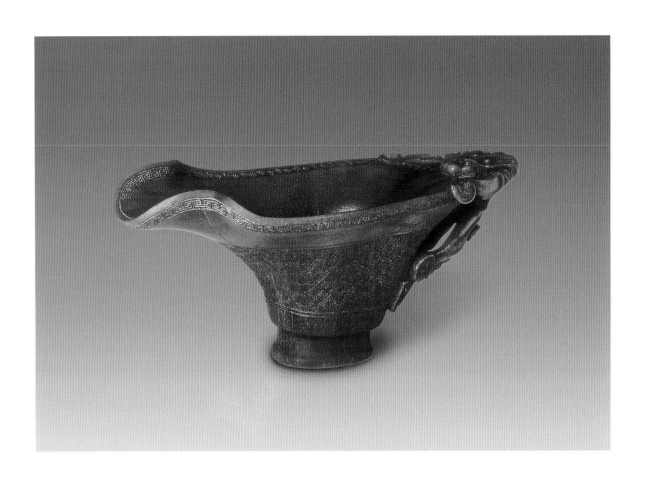

犀角服锦纹螭耳杯

清中期

犀角质

口径 10.5 ~ 18.3 厘米，足径 3.9 ~ 4.6 厘米，高 8 厘米

Rhinoceros Horn Cup with Dragon-shaped Handle and Brocade Patterns

Mid-Qing Dynasty

Rhinoceros Horn

Mouth Diameter 10.5-18.3 cm/ Foot Diameter 3.9-4.6 cm/ Height 8 cm

杯体稍矮，口沿敞开较大，内底浅，外壁剔刻连续锦地纹，杯耳镂雕螭龙形，抱杯沿，后腿分为二，变异为几何形式。其造型不同于一般的螭耳，是为配合杯身图案画的纹饰。

故宫博物院藏

The cup is slightly short, and has a bigger flared mouth and a shallow inner bottom. The exterior wall is decorated with successive brocade patterns. The handle is carved as a Chi-dragon shape in openwork. The dragon embraces the rim of the cup and its rear legs fall into two parts which are mutated into geometric patterns. Its shape is different from that of the ordinary Chi-dragon handle, which is for matching with the lines of the patterning on the body of the cup.

Preserved in The Palace Museum

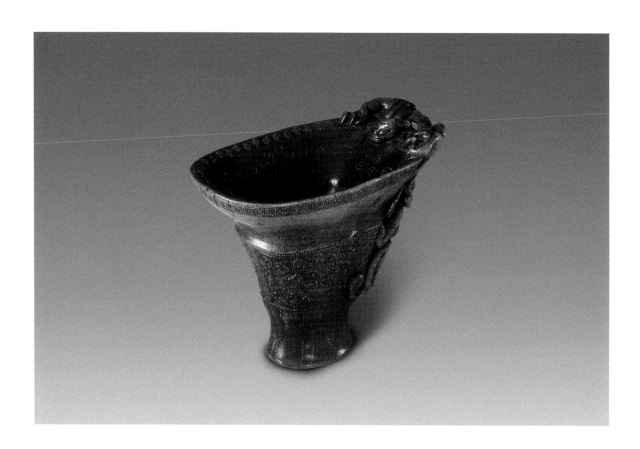

犀角雕饕餮蕉叶纹螭耳杯

清中期

犀角质

口径 8.2 ~ 13.5 厘米，足径 3.7 ~ 4.1 厘米，高 10.5 厘米

Rhinoceros Horn Cup Carved with Mystic Taotie, Banana Leaves and Dragon Designs

Mid-Qing Dynasty

Rhinoceros Horn

Mouth Diameter 8.2-13.5 cm/ Foot Diameter 3.7-4.1 cm/ Height 10.5 cm

杯身略呈扁圆，但不悖犀角本形。敞口，身较狭，高圈足微外撇。内口倾斜度较大，杯身内呈方形，浅底。杯口内外沿各装饰回纹一周，内口还阴刻变形"S"纹及云纹。外壁以回纹为地，剔刻饕餮纹，下饰蕉叶纹。耳为螭形，共镂雕三螭，大者鬃鬣贲张，探首杯内，如在窥视，一小螭攀于其身侧，另一小螭弯身在下。

故宫博物院藏

The cup is slightly oblate but still takes the natural form of the horn. The cup has a wide opening and a slender body. The high ring foot flares outward slightly and the internal opening slants greatly. The cup has a square and shallow bottom inside. The interior and exterior brims of the cup are decorated with circular meandering patterns, while the inner mouth is intaglioed with distorted S and cloud patterns. The exterior surface uses meandering pattern as its background and together with positively incised mystic Taotie and banana leaves patterns. The handle is carved in the form of a Chi-dragon. There are altogether three dragons carved in openwork. The big Chi-dragon is stretching its head excitedly as if peeping into the cup, with a smaller Chi-dragon climbing to its side while another smaller one bending its body below. Preserved in The Palace Museum

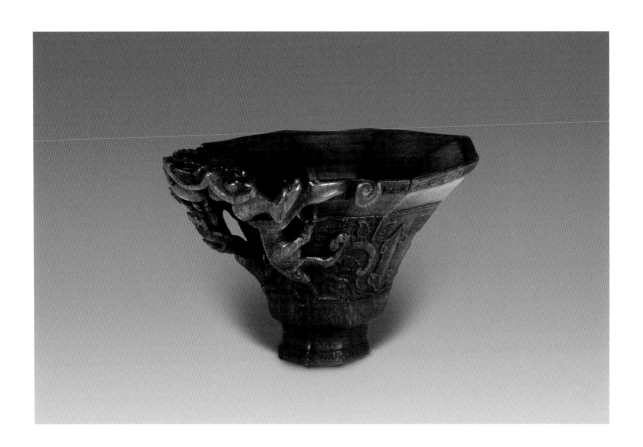

犀角雕双螭耳仿古兽面纹杯

清中期

犀角质

口径 8.5 ～ 13.6 厘米，足径 2.9 ～ 3.9 厘米，高 7.1 厘米

Rhinoceros Horn Cup Carved with Dragon Shaped Handles and Beast-face Images

Mid-Qing Dynasty

Rhinoceros Horn

Mouth Diameter 8.5-13.6 cm/ Foot Diameter 2.9-3.9 cm/ Height 7.1 cm

八方形，棕红色，敞口，撇足。雕双螭为柄，螭上身攀附在杯口，向杯内窥视，神态狡黠。杯身以阳文刻成庄严神秘的方夔兽面几何图案，口沿及底足阴刻回纹。

故宫博物院藏

The brownish red cup is octahedral and has a wide opening and a flared foot. The handle is carved with two Chi-dragons. With their upper bodies climbing and clinging to the cup rim, the two Chi-dragons, cunningly and lively, are stretching their heads as if peeping into the cup. Geometric designs of the solemn and mystic square kui-beast faces are carved in relief on the cup body, and the meandering pattern is carved in intaglio on the mouth rim and the foot.

Preserved in The Palace Museum

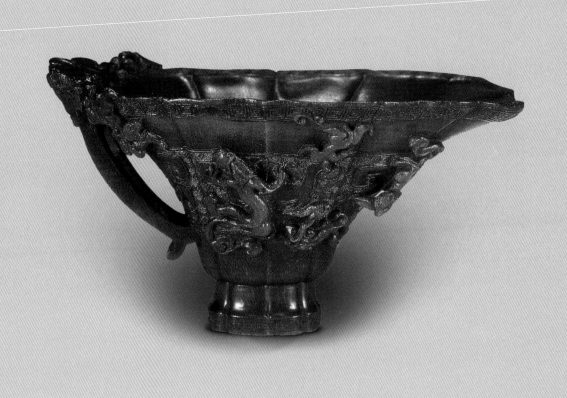

犀角雕兽纹柄仿古螭纹杯

清中期

犀角质

口径 10 ~ 17.5 厘米，足径 3.1 ~ 4.2 厘米，高 9.7 厘米

叶形，上阔下窄，朝天兽面耳。口沿及底足阴刻回纹，壁阴刻兽面锦地，锦地上饰九条攀爬的螭，形象生动，富有活力。

故宫博物院藏

Rhinoceros Horn Cup Carved with Beast-shaped Handle and Dragon Designs

Mid-Qing Dynasty

Rhinoceros Horn

Mouth Diameter 10–17.5 cm/ Foot Diameter 3.1–4.2 cm/ Height 9.7 cm

The cup takes the form of a leaf with a wide top and a narrow bottom. The handle is carved with a beast face design. Meandering patterns are carved in intaglio along the mouth rim and the foot. The body wall is carved with beast face patterns in intaglio as background. The background is decorated with nine Chi-dragons. The design is vivid, lifelike, and full of vitality.

Preserved in The Palace Museum

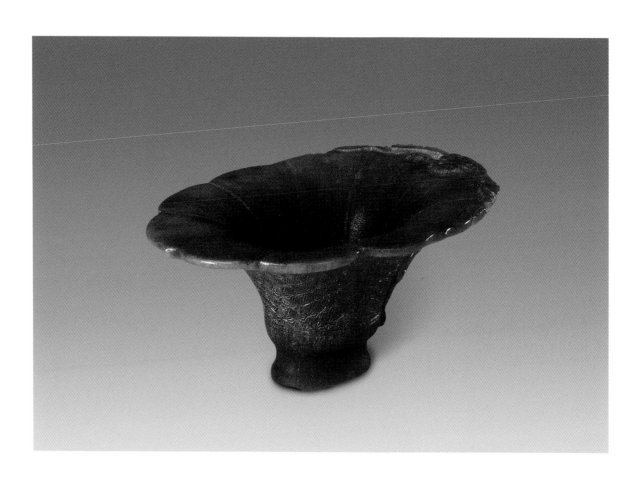

犀角雕螭纹杯

清中期

犀角质

口径 10.6 厘米，足径 4.9 厘米，高 3.5 厘米

Rhinoceros Horn Bowl Carved with Dragon Designs

Mid-Qing Dynasty

Rhinoceros Horn

Mouth Diameter 10.6 cm/ Foot Diameter 4.9 cm/ Height 3.5 cm

敞口，收腹，小玉璧底。壁较厚。外壁浮雕一周席纹地上，两夔龙纹相对，共三组。近口处有一周变体花叶纹，口沿上一周浅刻纹饰，亦甚别致，近足处有一周波浪纹。内壁打磨光滑，几可鉴人。

故宫博物院藏

The cup has a wide opening, a contracted body and a small jade wall base. The wall is thick. The background pattern of the exterior wall is a ring of storiform in relief with three pairs of double Kui-dragon designs face to face. There is a ring of varied flowers and leaf patterns near the rim, a ring of wave pattern near the foot and another ring of low relief pattern around the mouth rim with special ornamental effects. The inner wall of the cup is polished so smooth and shining that it can serve as a mirror.

Preserved in The Palace Museum

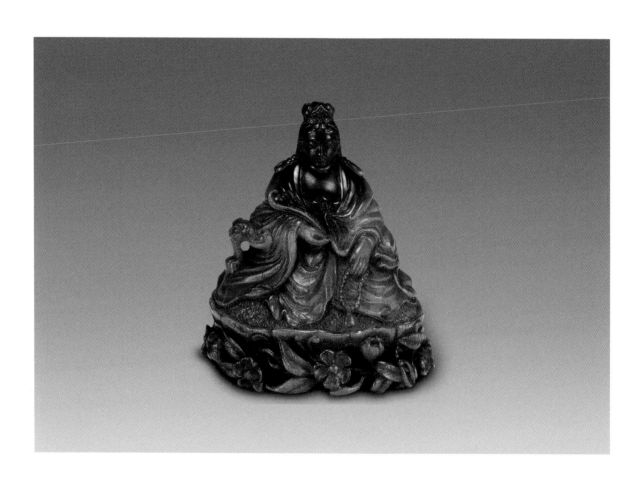

犀角雕桃花座观音

清中期

犀角质

底径 9 ~ 11.5 厘米，高 12.2 厘米

Rhinoceros Horn Statue Craved with Avalokitesvara Sitting on Peach Blossom Pedestal

Mid-Qing Dynasty

Rhinoceros horn

Bottom Diameter 9–11.5 cm/ Height 12.2 cm

广角制。染色。圆雕。观音头带发冠，身披广袖法衣，左手捏念珠，右手托如意，微闭双目，盘坐于花座之上。刻工细致，线条流畅，衣纹飘逸自然，表情细腻。

故宫博物院藏

The statue is made of African rhinoceros horn. It is a dyed circular engravure. With a hair headband crown and wearing wide sleeves vestments, holding prayer beads in her left hand and a ru-yi scepter in her right hand, the Avalokitesvara closes her eyes slightly and sits cross-legged on the peach blossom flower pedestal. The carving technique is fine and exquisite and the carved lines are smooth and flowing. With natural and elegant clothing lines, the facial expression is fine and smooth.

Preserved in The Palace Museum

象牙雕老人

清中期

象牙质

宽 5 厘米，高 15.5 厘米

立体圆雕，浅黄色。老人头挽发髻，身着束腰广袖长衫，倒背双手直立，昂首开口，面带微笑，向上观望。呈现出健康开朗之态。但垂胸长髯被切成弧线，显得死板，有工匠之气，是民间牙雕中的杰作。

故宫博物院藏

Ivory Statue with Carved Old Man

Mid-Qing Dynasty

Ivory

Width 5 cm/ Height 15.5 cm

The statue is a stereoscopic circular engravure in light yellow. The old man wears a tunic with wide sleeves, with his hair rolling up in a bun. Standing straightly with his hands clasping behind, the old man raises his head with mouth open, smiling and looking upward, which vividly shows that he is outgoing and in good health. But his long beard is cutting into unnatural and stiff curves. However it was still a masterpiece of ivory statues at the time.

Preserved in The Palace Museum

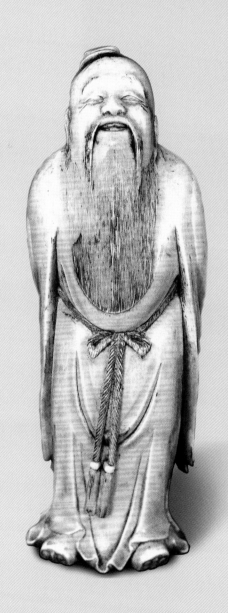

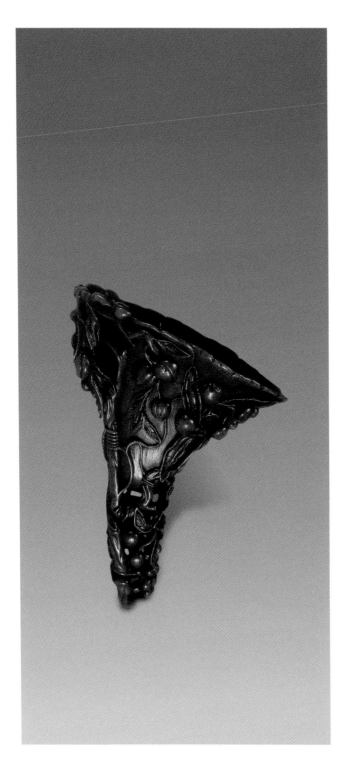

犀角雕果实杯

清中期

犀角质

口径 11 ~ 17.7 厘米，高 21 厘米

Rhinoceros Horn Cup Carved with Fruits

Mid-Qing Dynasty

Rhinoceros Horn

Mouth Diameter 11-17.7 cm/ Height 21 cm

该藏由非洲犀牛额前角随天然形状镂雕而成。
棕色。上宽下尖，宽流。采用镂刻浮雕技法，
通体刻葡萄、寿桃、石榴、枇杷等，须藤萦绕，
枝壮叶阔，硕果累累。

故宫博物院藏

The cup is engraved in openwork with the
natural shape of the anterior part of the African
rhinoceros horn. The cup is brown and has a
broad top, a pointed bottom and a broad spout.
The whole cup is carved in high relief. The
entire cup is engraved with designs of grapes,
peaches, pomegranates and loquats. With
intertwined vines and tendrils, big branches
and thick leaves, the carved trees are full of
countless rich fruits.

Preserved in The Palace Museum

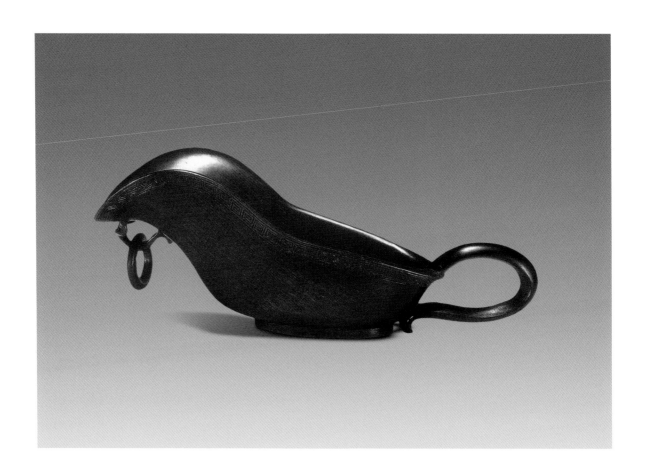

犀角雕仿古光素匜

清中期

犀角质

长 17 厘米，宽 8 厘米，高 9.6 厘米

Rhinoceros Horn Bailer with Antique Looking in Plain Color

Mid-Qing Dynasty

Rhinoceros Horn

Length 17 cm/ Width 8 cm/ Height 9.6 cm

浅棕色，椭圆圈足。采用浅渴热熔法，将匜身做成光素体，衬以阴线回纹口沿，匜前流口下嵌镶有夔耳活环，在匜柄外嵌有较深的圈把。造型奇特优美，莹润细腻，是犀角中较为少见、难得的珍品。

故宫博物院藏

The bailer is light brown and has an elliptical ring foot. The bright plain body was made through the heat fusion method. The mouth edge is incised with geometric shade lines. Below the head part of the spout it is inlaid with a movable hoop in the shape of a kui-dragon. On the exterior of the bailer it is inlaid with a deep ring becket. The bailer is shaped singularly and gracefully. With exquisite, bright and smooth surface, it is really a rare treasure.

Preserved in The Palace Museum

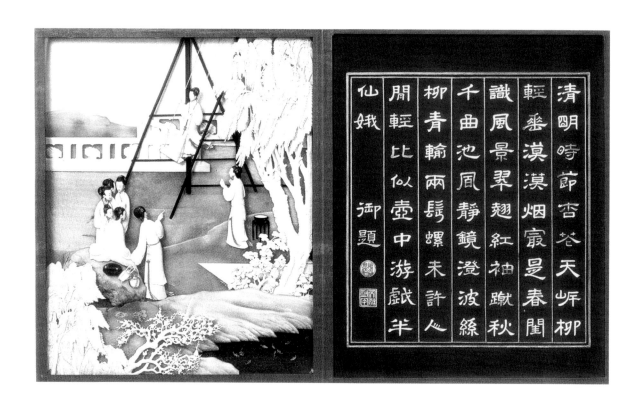

清明時節杏苔天㭊柳
輕毵漠漠烟宸是春閨
識風景翠翹紅袖蹴秋
千曲池凮靜鏡澄波絲
柳青輸兩鬌螺未許人
閒輕比似壺中游戲半
仙娥　御題

象牙雕杨柳秋千图

清中期

象牙质

长 39.1 厘米，宽 32.9 厘米，厚 3.2 厘米

为《月曼清游》册中三月景。园中垂柳桃树旁，秋千架高耸，一女正在愉快地荡秋千，七女在架下或立或坐昂首观看，似乎正在为她数着荡数。右方嵌螺钿隶书七律一首，诗中写道："清明时节杏花天，岸柳轻垂漠漠烟。最是春闺识风景，翠翘红袖蹴秋千。曲池风静镜澄波，丝柳青输两鬓螺。未许人闲轻比似，壶中游戏半仙娥。"诗后钤"得思""千秋坚固"二印。

故宫博物院藏

Ivory Carving Designs with Women Having a Swing under Poplar and Willow Tree

Mid-Qing Dynasty

Ivory

Length 39.1 cm/ Width 32.9 cm/ Thickness 3.2 cm

The carving depicts the March scenery in the book of Yue Man Qing You. A swing is set up highly beside willow and peach trees in the garden. A lady is merrily having a swing and another seven ladies sitting or standing under the frame are looking up at her as if counting the swinging numbers for her. A poem, which was written by the Emperor Qianlong about the scenery of March and happiness of ladies, is carved on the right side of the design in official script with mother-of-pearl inlay. Two official seals are stamped at the end of the poem which read "De Si" and "Qian Qiu Jian Gu".

Preserved in The Palace Museum

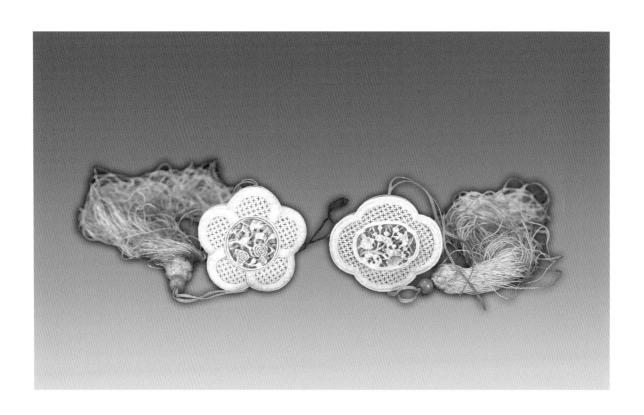

象牙雕花鸟香盒

清中期

象牙质

左：高 1.8 厘米，径 3.2 ~ 4 厘米

右：高 1.6 厘米，径 3.8 厘米

Ivory Pomanders Carved with Designs of Birds and Flowers

Mid-Qing Dynasty

Ivory

The Left One: Height 1.8 cm/ Diameter 3.2–4 cm

The Right One: Height 1.6 cm/ Diameter 3.8 cm

一呈海棠花形，一呈梅花形，均以镂刻染色
技法制成。小盒从中分启，周缘微薄，中间
鼓起，上下重叠较深，有明黄色绦带从孔中
穿过，绦带下端束有珊瑚米珠及彩线丝穗。
小盒通体镂刻万字纹，中间刻以花鸟纹。

故宫博物院藏

One box is in the shape of a begonia, and the
other one is in the shape of a quincunx. Both
are made in staining techniques and openwork.
The rim of the boxes is a bit thin and the central
part is bulging, with overlaps up and down. A
brilliant yellow silk braid is threading through
the hole of the box. The lower part of the silk
braid is corral beads and colorful tassels. The
whole box is engraved with swastika pattern,
with birds and flower patterns among them.
Preserved in The Palace Museum

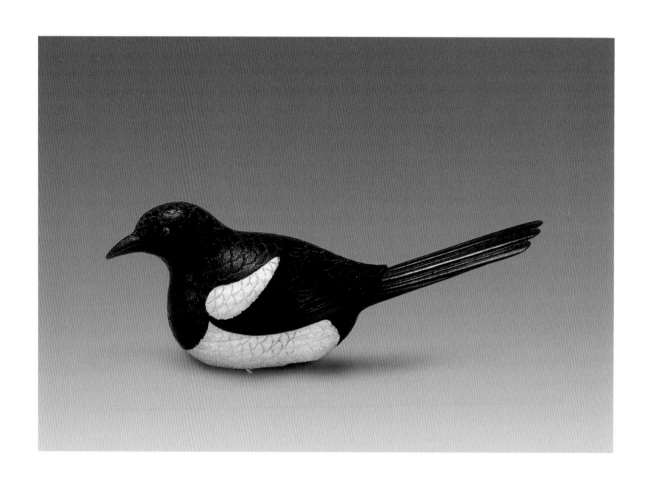

染牙喜鹊盒

清中期

象牙质

长 12 厘米，宽 4.5 厘米，高 5.6 厘米

Ivory Box Dyed and Carved in the Shape of Magpie

Mid-Qing Dynasty

Ivory

Length 12 cm/ Width 4.5 cm/ Height 5.6 cm

圆雕。卧鸟式，长尾后翘，尖嘴，圆睛，白翅，白腹，黑爪缩于腹下。盒于鸟身中间上、下分启，上半身为盖，盖口处翅羽交错，外观无接痕。此盒造型精巧典雅，色泽自然。

故宫博物院藏

The box is a circular carving. It is in the shape of a crouching bird whose long tail is tip-tilted. The bird has a sharp and pointed beak, round eyes, white wings, white belly and black claws under its belly. The box is divided into two parts along the middle part of the body. The upper part of the body serves as the lid and the exterior circumferential joint between the two parts is not easy to be seen due to its intervening feather and wing patterns at the mouth part. This box is exquisite and elegant in shape and natural in color and luster.

Preserved in The Palace Museum

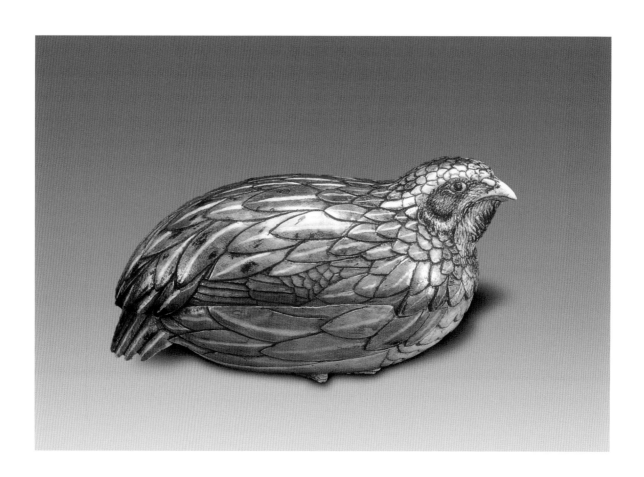

染牙鹌鹑盒

清中期

象牙质

长 12 厘米，宽 4.5 厘米，高 5.6 厘米

Ivory Box Dyed and Carved in the Shape of Quail

Mid-Qing Dynasty

Ivory

Length 12 cm/ Width 4.5 cm/ Height 5.6 cm

圆雕。蹲伏状，背与头部为盖。尖嘴，眼直视，双尾下垂，三爪足踡缩于腹下。头部刻鳞纹，眼睛周围绒毛疏密，身上分层次雕成叶形羽，由浅入深染成棕色。

故宫博物院藏

The box is a circular carving. It is in the shape of a crouching bird. The bird's back and head serve as the lid. It has a sharp beak, straight looking eyes, and drooping tail. The three-jaw feet huddle up under its belly. The head part is engraved with scale ripple patterns, and fine hairs are around the eyes. The body is carved in layers with feathers of leaf shapes, and dyed from light to dark brown.

Preserved in The Palace Museum

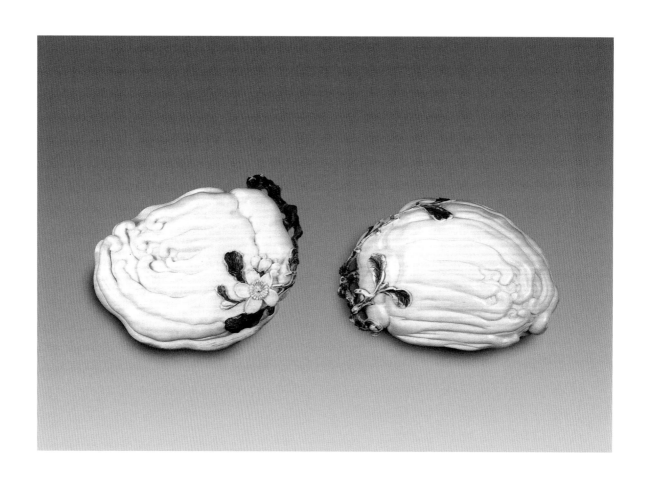

染牙佛手式盒

清中期

象牙质

长 9.5 厘米，宽 7 厘米，高 2.8 厘米

Ivory Box Dyed and Carved in the Shape of Finger Citron

Mid-Qing Dynasty

Ivory

Length 9.5 cm/ Width 7 cm/ Height 2.8 cm

圆雕。盒身正反两面所刻佛手呈象牙自然色，
在果蒂处用染色和高浮雕技法刻成褐枝、绿
叶、粉花及花蕾。

故宫博物院藏

The box is a circular carving. Both sides of
the box are engraved with finger citron in the
natural ivory color, while at the pedicel, brown
branches, green leaves, pink flowers and buds
are dyed and carved in high relief techniques.

Preserved in The Palace Museum

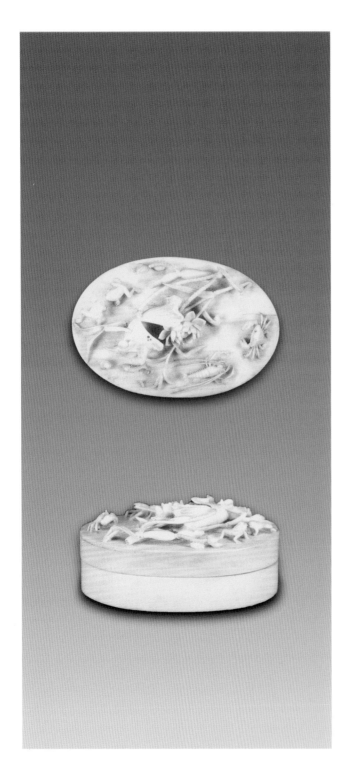

象牙雕荷花椭圆小盒

清中期

象牙质

径 3.8 ~ 5.8 厘米，高 2.5 厘米

Small Ivory Oval Box Carved with Lotus Pattern

Mid-Qing Dynasty

Ivory

Diameter 3.8–5.8 cm/ Height 2.5 cm

在壁薄如纸的象牙小盒盖面上，精心雕有荷花、莲藕、蛙、蟹、虾等物。盒内正中有一活环小水罐，一条活环小链与盖相接，小罐四周分布有叶形小盘与白藕一支，盘中盛佛手和菱角，一只蜘蛛正向水罐爬去。在盒盖内面，一群蚂蚁正在搬运一只仰卧的蝇虫。

故宫博物院藏

The surface of the tiny ivory box lid is as thin as paper, and it is decorated with carefully carved lotus root, frog, crab, and shrimps etc. There is a tiny water pot with a movable link in the center of the box, and a small movable chain connects with the lid. A lotus root and a leaf-shaped tiny plate are around the pot, in addition to finger citron, water chestnut, and a spider crawling towards the pot. Inside the lid, a group of ants are moving a supine fly.

Preserved in The Palace Museum

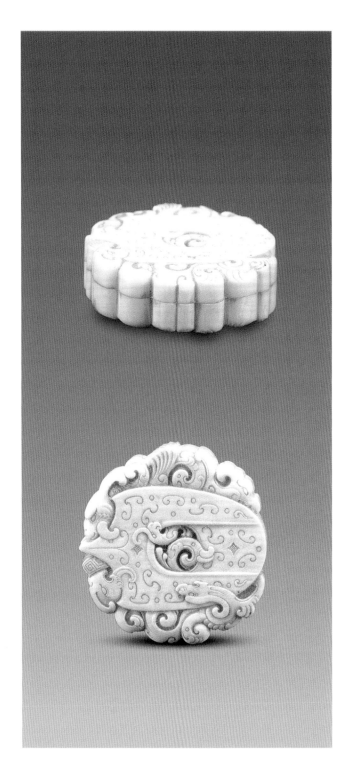

象牙雕玉琶式盒

清中期

象牙质

高 1.6 厘米

Ivory Box Carved with Jade Pa Design

Mid-Qing Dynasty

Ivory

Height 1.6 cm

仿战国璧，盒内有螺旋扣钮。盒面两端以阳

文浅浮雕双夔龙，使小盒正反两面都可作为

盒面。图案布局严谨规整，刀法细腻流畅，

是清中期小型牙雕摆设中的佳品。

故宫博物院藏

The box is an imitation of the Warring States
jade disc. There is a turnbuckle and knob inside
the box. Two kui-dragon images are carved
in low relief at both ends of the box surface
so that the inner and outer surfaces of the box
can be used as the obverse side. The overall
arrangement of the images is precise and
orderly. The carving skills are fine and smooth.
It was a masterpiece of small ivory carvings
for furnishing and decoration in the Mid-Qing
Dynasty.

Preserved in The Palace Museum

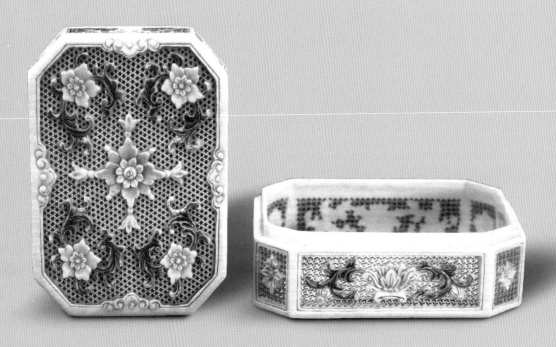

染牙镂雕花卉长方折角盒

清中期

象牙质

长 7.6 厘米，宽 5.4 厘米，高 3 厘米

银白色，长方折角形，为一整块象牙掏刻而成。盒从中分启，上下各八个框，框中通体镂钻万字锦纹地，锦地上分别浮刻染色勾莲宝相花卉纹。盖面四周刻有如意边缘，中间钻环钱纹锦地，锦地上对称浮雕蕃枝花卉及出脊宝相花纹。

故宫博物院藏

Dyed-ivory Rectangular Bevel Box with Engraved Flowers in Openwork

Mid-Qing Dynasty

Ivory

Length 7.6 cm/ Width 5.4 cm/ Height 3 cm

The silver white box is rectangle and beveled. The box is engraved from a single piece of ivory. The box is separated from the central section into the upper and lower parts, each with 8 frames. All the frames are engraved with the swastika background patterns, and the rosette pattern is dyed and carved respectively in relief. Ruyi scepter pattern is carved all around the edge of the lid, with hollow rings and coin designs as background patterns. The thriving branches and ridged rosette patterns are symmetrically carved in relief on the lid.

Preserved in The Palace Museum

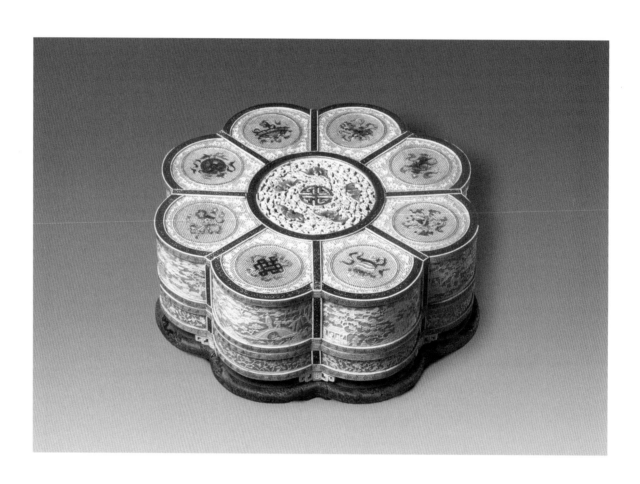

象牙镂空山水八瓣式盒

清中期

象牙质

直径 39.6 厘米，高 12.8 厘米

Ivory Box of Eight Petal Shape Carved with Landscape Patterns in Openwork

Mid-Qing Dynasty

Ivory

Diameter 39.6 cm/ Height 12.8 cm

呈八瓣梅花形，匠人采用拼镶、拨镂、透刻技法，以对称的组合方式制成。盒面和盒壁用拨镂染色方法，均以蓝色梅花锦纹作为边框。盒盖是中圆呈放射的八瓣花式面，用钻刻技法，通刻梅纹锦地，用浅雕、染色技法，在中圆内刻有五幅捧寿云纹图案。

故宫博物院藏

The box is shaped as a plum blossom with 8 petals. The craftsman employed a symmetric combination method to fit the parts together with the skills of inlaying, ivory dyeing, carving and openwork. With blue plum-blossom background patterns as the frames, the surface of the cover and the box walls are dyed and engraved. The box cover is shaped as an eight-petal face in radial pattern with a circle section at the center through the boring and carving techniques. Covered with engraved plum-blossom patterns, the central circle section is dyed and carved in low relief with a cloud pattern of luckiness and longevity.

Preserved in The Palace Museum

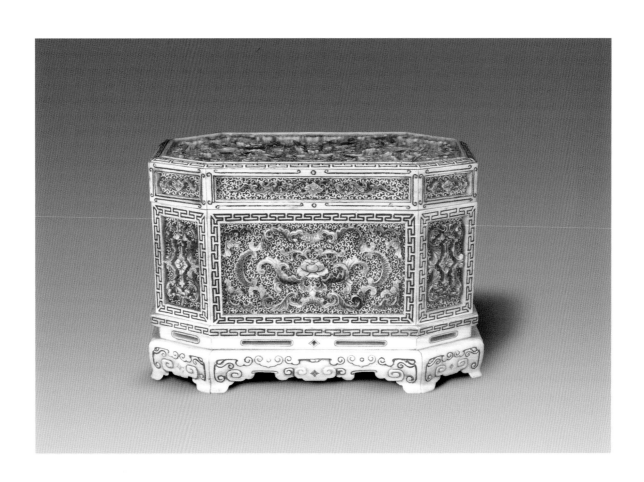

象牙镂空花卉长方盒

清中期

象牙质

长 14.8 厘米，宽 7.6 厘米，高 10 厘米

Ivory Rectangular Box Carved with Flowers and Plants Patterns in Openwork

Mid-Qing Dynasty

Ivory

Length 14.8 cm/ Width 7.6 cm/ Height 10 cm

采用拨镂、染色、镂钻等多种技法将 42 块大小不同的牙片拼镶而成。盒盖、盒体以阴刻雷纹为边框，框内八面开光，通体镂钻勾莲锦纹地，锦地上对称浮雕染色蕾枝莲花纹，枝叶挺括，舒朗精美。盒体下连有填彩流云纹八足座。

故宫博物院藏

The box is put together and inlaid with forty-two different sized pieces of ivory through various techniques such as ivory dyeing, carving, boring and engraving, etc. Thunder patterns are carved in intaglio as frames of the cover and the body of the box with open light on all eight sides. The entire box is engraved with lotus and mosaic patterns. Bright and elegant, the lotus buds patterns are dyed and carved symmetrically in relief on the brocade with stiff and smooth branches and leaves. The box connects the eight legs base with colored cloud patterns.

Preserved in The Palace Museum

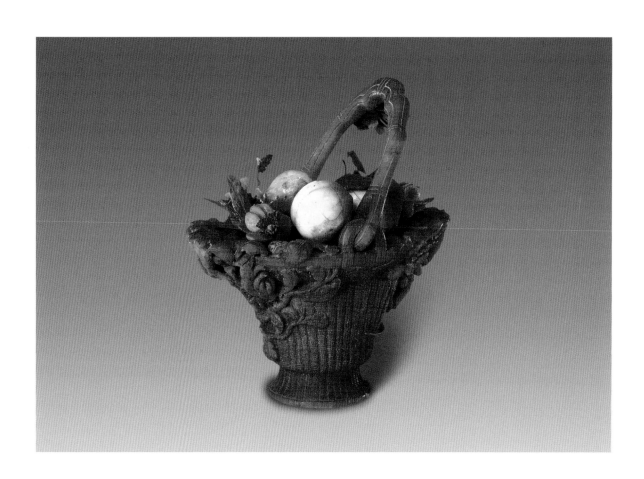

犀角雕花篮

清中期

犀角质

足径 5 厘米，高 16.5 厘米

Rhinoceros Horn Basket Carved with Flowers

Mid-Qing Dynasty

Rhinoceros Horn

Foot Diameter 5 cm/ Height 16.5 cm

花篮形。外壁满雕竹篾编织状纹饰，非常精细。口沿处浮雕佛手、玉兰、向日葵、灵芝等花果及枝叶，并镂雕提梁。篮内以染牙、宝石等配合金属丝制枝条，表现各色花叶，如玉兰、菊、石竹、桃子等。

故宫博物院藏

The item is shaped as a flower basket. The exterior wall of the flower basket is completely carved with very fine interlaced patterns of bamboo strips. Various flowers and fruits, including fingered citrons, yulan magnolias, sunflowers and lucid ganoderma, are carved in relief along the rim of the basket, and the handle is engraved in openwork. Inside the basket, the metal wire twigs together with the dyed ivories and jewels represent flowers and leaves of all kinds, such as yulan magnolia, chrysanthemum, dianthus, and peach.

Preserved in The Palace Museum

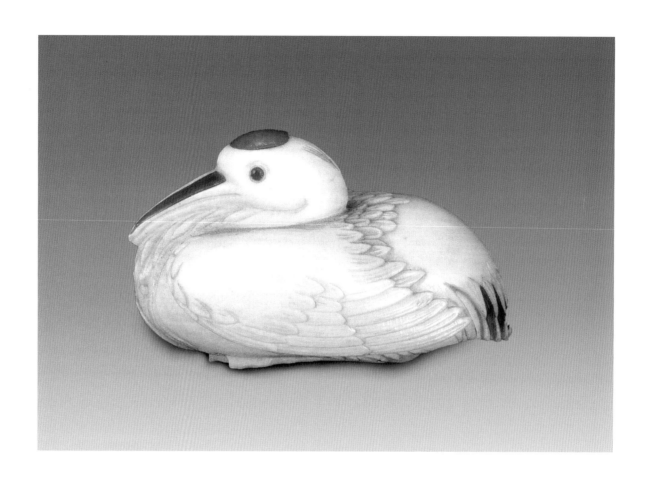

象牙仙鹤形鼻烟壶

清中期

象牙质

长 4.7 厘米，腹宽 2.9 厘米

Ivory Snuff Bottle in the Shape of Red-crowned Crane

Mid-Qing Dynasty

Ivory

Length 4.7 cm/ Belly Width 2.9 cm

圆雕。烟壶呈伏卧丹顶鹤形。器身白色，鹤喙上部、双眼、尾部飞羽嵌玳瑁，头顶上鲜红的肉冠嵌鸡血石，双腿染为绿色。颈下有盖，设有暗销，盖内阴刻篆文"乾隆年制"四字款。盖内下连象牙勺。本物是宫廷造办处牙匠为乾隆帝精心设计的巧雕之作。

故宫博物院藏

The snuff bottle is a circular carving. It is shaped as a prone red-crowned crane. The bottle itself is white; the top of the beak, its eyes and tail are inlaid with hawksbill shell. The bright red caruncle is inlaid with bloodstone, and the legs are ivory dyed in green. A lid with a dowel is under the neck. A seal script is incised in intaglio at the inner part of the lid which reading "Qian Long Nian Zhi" means it was made during the reign of Qianlong. An ivory spoon is attached to the lid inside. This item was an artful masterpiece well-designed and engraved for Qianlong Emperor by the craftsman in the Royal Court Workshops.

Preserved in The Palace Museum

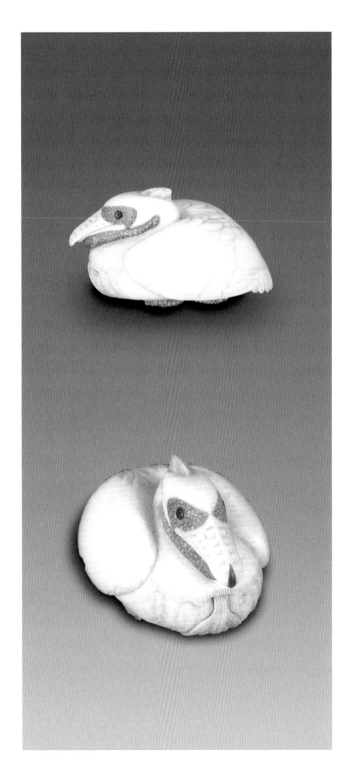

象牙鱼鹰形鼻烟壶

清中期

象牙质

长 4.8 厘米，腹宽 2.9 厘米

Ivory Snuff Bottle in the Shape of Osprey

Mid-Qing Dynasty

Ivory

Length 4.8 cm/ Belly width 2.9 cm

圆雕。烟壶呈鱼鹰伏卧形。器身白色，双眼与嘴尖上部嵌玳瑁，眼睛四周、颈下、双腿雕刻棕色颗粒状装饰。鱼鹰体羽丰满，喙尖而钩曲，头上生白丝状羽。颈下有盖，设有暗销，盖内阴刻篆文"乾隆年制"四字款。盖内下连象牙勺。本壶是宫廷造办处牙匠为乾隆帝精心制作的御用之物。

故宫博物院藏

The snuff bottle is a circular carving. It is shaped as a prone osprey. The bottle itself is white; its eyes and the upper part of its beak are inlaid with hawksbill shells. The carved brown granular decoration is all around its eyes, the underneath of the neck and its legs. The osprey has plenty body feathers, and its hooked beak is sharp. Its head is covered with white filamentous feather. A lid with a dowel is under the neck. A seal script is incised in intaglio at the inner part of the lid which reads "Qian Long Nian Zhi" means it was made during the reign of Qianlong. An ivory spoon is attached to the lid inside. This item was an artful masterpiece well-designed and engraved for Qianlong Emperor by the craftsman in the Royal Court Workshops. Preserved in The Palace Museum

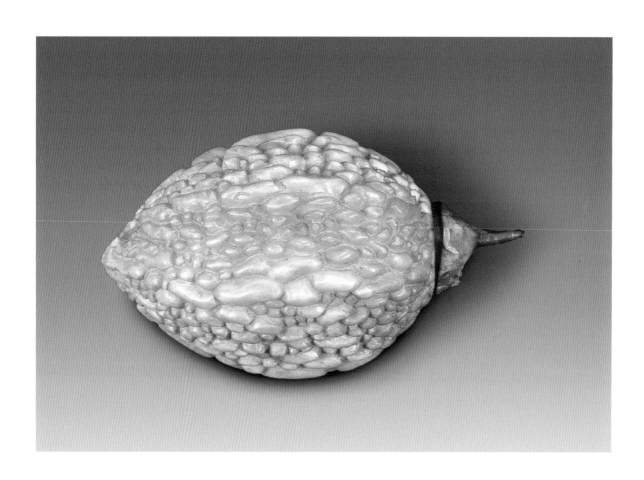

象牙雕苦瓜形鼻烟壶

清中期

象牙质

长 7 厘米，腹宽 3.8 厘米

Ivory Snuff Bottle in the Shape of Bitter Gourd

Mid-Qing Dynasty

Ivory

Length 7 cm/ Belly Width 3.8 cm

圆雕。黄赤色。此器为纺锤形，表面有瘤状
突起，并有六道棱，瓜蒂作盖，仿叶掌状，
为绿色染牙。

故宫博物院藏

The golden bottle is a circular carving and is
shaped as a spindle. The bottle surface is carved
with strumae and six arris. The muskmelon
pedicel which is in the shape of a leaf is utilized
as the lid. It is dyed in green color.

Preserved in The Palace Museum

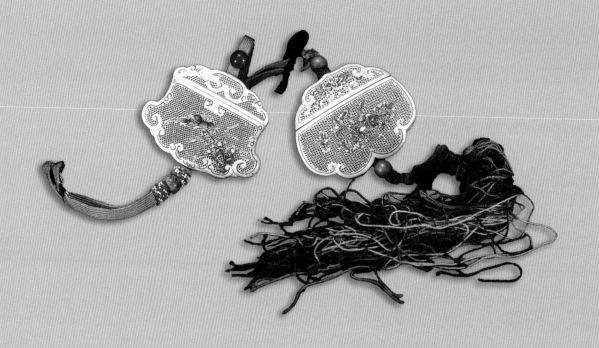

染牙镂雕花卉火镰套

清中期

象牙质

长 7 厘米，宽 5.6 厘米

斧形、扁锁形。均镂钻古钱纹锦地，锦地上又以浅浮雕及染色技法刻有石榴、佛手、兰花等花果图案。造型新颖，玲珑生动，纹饰既严谨又活泼。出自官廷造办处如意馆技师之手。

故宫博物院藏

Dyed Ivory Flint Cover with Engraved Flowers in Openwork

Mid-Qing Dynasty

Ivory

Length 7 cm/ Width 5.6 cm

The cover is shaped as an axe or a flat lock. The whole surface is engraved with ancient coin patterns, on which flowers and fruits are dyed and carved in low relief, including pomegranate, fingered citron and orchid. With innovative designs and exquisite patterns, the emblazonry is not only precise but also vivid. These crafts were made by craftsman from Ruyi House in the Royal Court Workshop.

Preserved in The Palace Museum

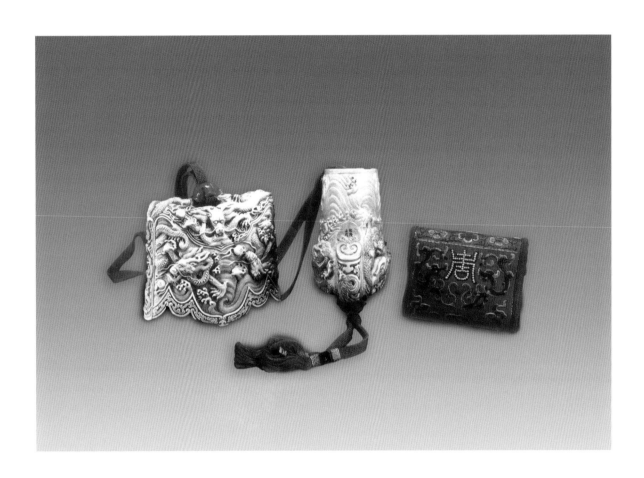

象牙雕海水云龙火镰套

清中期

象牙质

长 11.2 厘米，宽 5.9 厘米

Ivory Flint Cover Carved with Seawater Patterns and Designs of Clouds and Dragons

Mid-Qing Dynasty

Ivory

Length 11.2 cm/ Width 5.9 cm

覆钟式，平面光素底，内有明黄丝套盛装火石、火镰及引火绒纸。整个套盒由一条黄丝带从中穿连，上端由一珊瑚珠固定开启，下端由一染牙荷叶结托。

故宫博物院藏

The covers are shaped as bells. The bottom is flat and plain. The inside of the cover is a bright yellow silk bag full of fire-stones, flints and tinder. The whole box is connected in the middle with a yellow silk ribbon. The upper part is a fixed coral bead to open and close the box, and the bottom is a dyed ivory lotus leaf knot.

Preserved in The Palace Museum

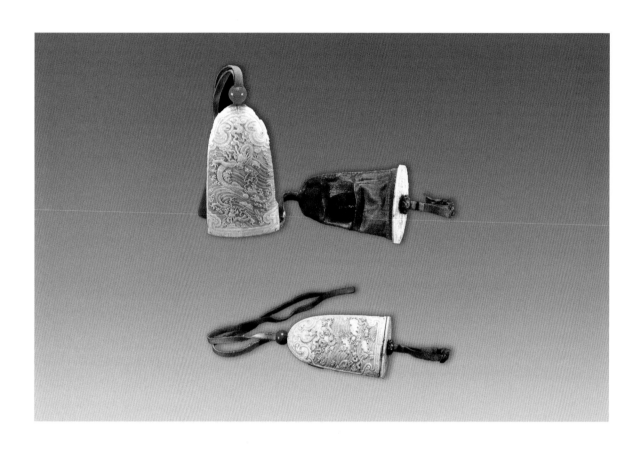

黄振效象牙雕海水云龙火镰套

清中期

象牙质

长 8 厘米，宽 7.4 厘米

Ivory Flint Cover Carved with Seawater Patterns and Designs of Clouds and Dragons By Huang Zhenxiao

Mid-Qing Dynasty

Ivory

Length 8 cm/ Width 7.4 cm

形如荷包，是宫廷象牙雕刻家黄振效于 1742 年制作的。他按照清宫服饰的要求，将一块实体象牙套剖成两部分，上为盖，下为盒，中空，出一根黄丝带及两块莲叶形的珊瑚饰珠穿连，并采用深浅浮雕技法。

故宫博物院藏

The cover is shaped as a lotus pouch. It was made in 1742 by Huang Zhenxiao, an ivory craftsman in the royal court. Based on the requirements of official costume in Qing Dynasty, he dissected a piece of solid ivory into two parts and then hollowed each of them: the upper part as lid and the bottom part as box. A yellow silk rope with two lotus-leaf shaped coral beads connects the two parts, and the cover is carved with patterns in high and low relief.

Preserved in The Palace Museum

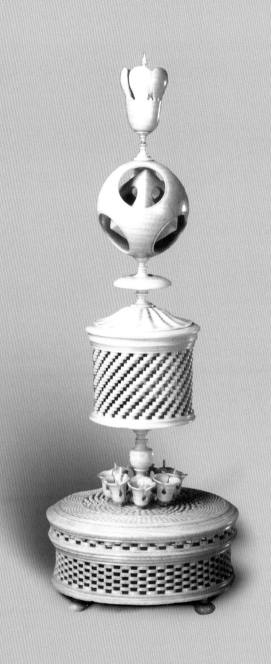

象牙雕套盒

清末

象牙质

高 21 厘米

可分上、中、下三部分，每部分均可拆卸，上层为镂空六孔圆球，内有一方体，亦六孔，空心。中纳骰子，有一至六点，黑漆点成。中、下二部为一高一扁二圆盒，均可分开为盖、身。装饰虚实方格或斜垒方格纹，灵感似来自编织物。或用以储物，或放置香料。

故宫博物院藏

Carved Ivory Coffret

Late Qing Dynasty

Ivory

Height 21 cm

The set are divided into top, middle and bottom sections, with each part detachable. The top section which has 6 holes in openwork is a round ball. Inside the round ball there is a cubic part which also has 6 hollow holes. There is a dice in the cubic part with carved numbers 1 to 6 in black paint. The middle and bottom sections are two round boxes, one tall, one short and both are separable. The boxes are decorated with empty and solid square patterns or oblique grid patterns. The inspiration of this craftsmanship is likely from the weaving products. The set was utilized either for storing things or storing spices.

Preserved in The Palace Museum

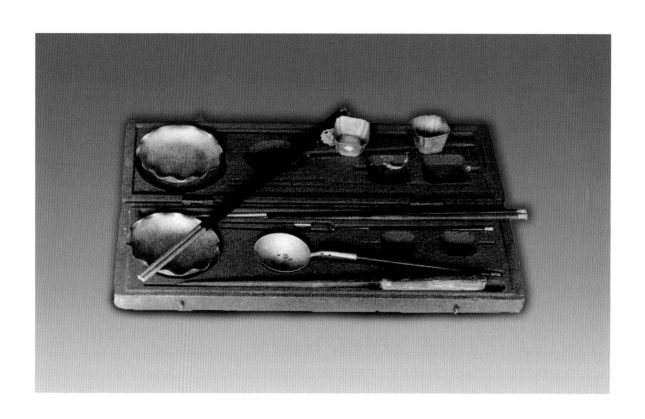

盒装餐具

清末

银质、木质

盒：长 33.1 厘米，宽 11.2 厘米

木箸：长 30 厘米，直径 0.25~0.45 厘米

Box-packed Tableware

Late Qing Dynasty

Silvery and Wood

Box: Length 33.1 cm/ Width 11.2 cm

Wood chopsticks: Length 30 cm/ Diameter 0.25 -0.45 cm

盒内两面均旋控雕刻出对应的圆形、方形及长条形凹槽，以盛装不同形状的餐具。盒内共有镶银木箸2双、银质木柄小勺1把、木柄餐刀1把、银盘2件、银方杯2只及果叉1把。其中木箸系用黑檀木制成，两端镶银，整体呈圆柱形，形态修长匀称，制作精美。多种用具装入一盒后井然有序，在密封状态下卫生洁净。

中国箸文化陈列馆藏

Different shapes of partitions are carved on both sides of the box, including round, square and rectangular shapes, for placing different tableware. The box contains nine pieces of tableware: two pairs of wood chopsticks with silver inlay, one small silver spoon with a wooden handle, one knife with a wooden handle, two silver plates, two square silver cups and one fruit fork. The wood chopsticks are made of black wood, and both ends are inlaid with silver. Cylindrical and slender, the chopsticks are exquisite in making. Various utensils are enclosed in it orderly, clean and healthy in sealed conditions.

Preserved in Chinese Chopsticks Culture Museum

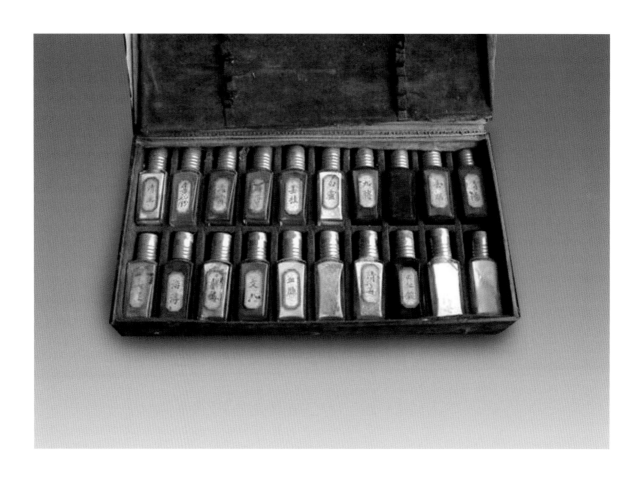

出诊药包

清末

木质、玻璃质

长 33 厘米，宽 17.7 厘米，厚 4.4 厘米

Medicine Package for Home Visit

Modern Times

Wood and Glass

Length 33 cm/ Width 17.7 cm/ Thickness 4.4 cm

为清末丹阳名医贺季衡使用。贺氏晚年以"指禅"名其斋，自号"指禅老人"。

江苏省中医药博物馆藏

This package was utilized by a famous doctor whose name was He Jihen in the late Qing Dynasty in Danyang. Mr. He Jihen named his study "Zhi Chan" in his late life, so he called himself "Zhi Chan Lao Ren", meaning an old man who lived in Zhi Chan study.

Preserved in Jiangsu Museum of Traditional Chinese Medicine

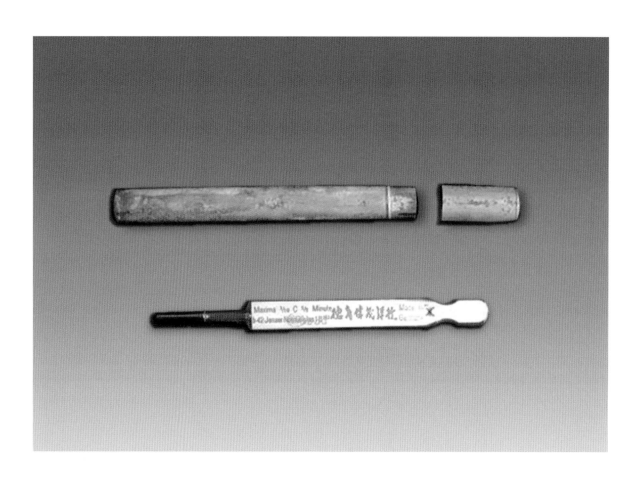

体温表

清末

玻璃质

长 12.8 厘米

Thermometer

Modern Times

Glass

Length 12.8 cm

为清末丹阳名医贺季衡（晚年以"指禅"名
其斋，自号"指禅老人"）使用。

江苏省中医药博物馆藏

The thermometer was utilized by a famous
doctor whose name was He Jihen in the late
Qing Dynasty in Danyang. Mr. He Jihen named
his study "Zhi Chan" in his late life, so he
called himself "Zhi Chan Lao Ren", meaning an
old man who lived in Zhi Chan study.
Preserved in Jiangsu Museum of Traditional
Chinese Medicine

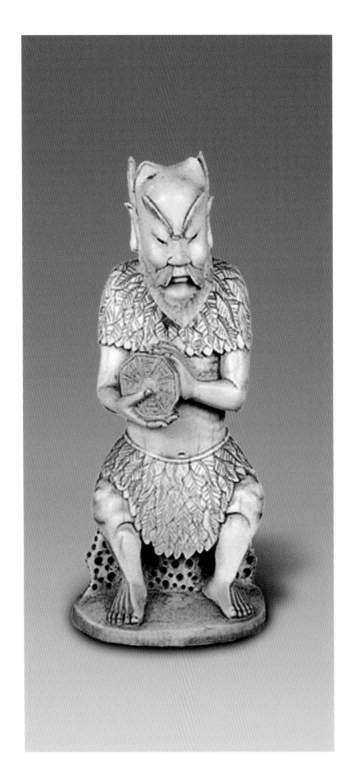

伏羲像

清

象牙质

座宽 7.5 厘米，通高 19 厘米

Fuxi Statue

Qing Dynasty

Ivory

Pedestal Width 7.5 cm/ Height 19 cm

皇甫谧在《帝王世纪》中云："伏羲画八卦所以六气六府，五行五脏，阴阳四时，水火升降，得以有象；百病之理，得以有类。乃尝百药而制九针，以拯夭枉焉。"此像坐视，双手持八卦，赤脚，树叶做衣。

上海中医药博物馆藏

This is a sitting statue of Fuxi, the first of the Three Sovereigns in ancient China. Fuxi is bare-footed, and he is wearing clothes made of tree leaves and holding the Eight Diagrams in his both hands. In the book *Ages of Kings*, the author Huangpu Mi said: Fuxi created the Eight Diagrams which reflect the basic principles of people's organs and how they function so that people can recognize the causes of hundreds of diseases. Fuxi, therefore, tasted hundreds of herb medicines and invented nine needles to save people from dying young.
Preserved in Shanghai Museum of Traditional Chinese Medicine

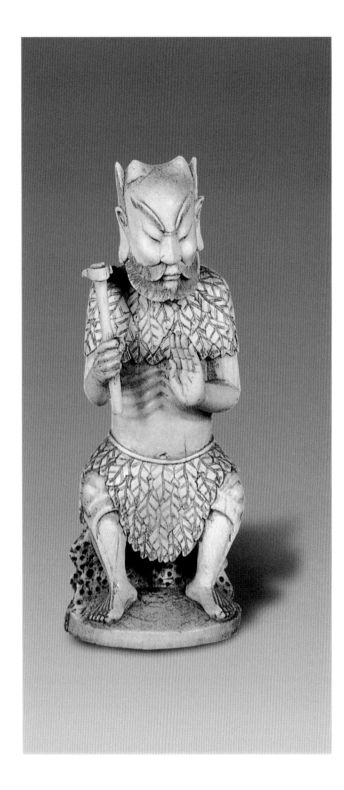

黄帝像

清

象牙质

座宽 8 厘米，通高 18.5 厘米

Statue of Yellow Emperor

Qing Dynasty

Ivory

Pedestal Width 8 cm/ Height 18.5 cm

黄帝为传说中的中华民族的先祖，亦传为中国医药学的创始人之一。《黄帝内经》就是托其名的医著。

上海中医药博物馆藏

The Yellow Emperor was the legendary progenitor of Chinese nation who was also said to be one of the cofounders of traditional Chinese medicine. *Huangdi Neijing*, a very famous medical book in ancient China, got its name from him.

Preserved in Shanghai Museum of Traditional Chinese Medicine

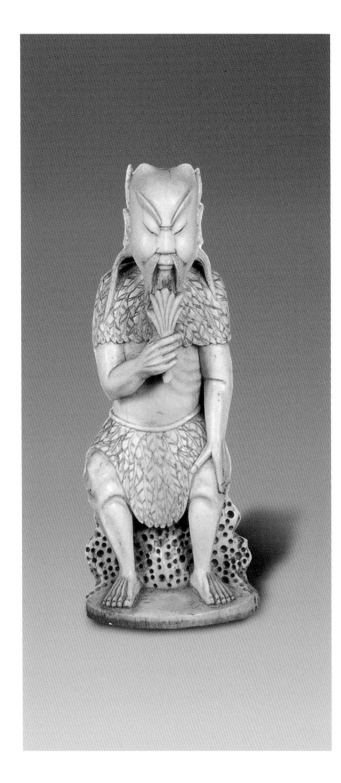

神农像

清

象牙质

座宽 7.5 厘米, 通高 19 厘米

Shengnong Statue

Qing Dynasty

Ivory

Pedestal Width 7.5 cm/ Height 19 cm

手持草，作品尝状，与"神农尝百草，始创医药"

的记载相符。

上海中医药博物馆藏

It is a statue of Shengnong, the inventor of Chinese medicine, tasting herb medicine in his hand, which tallies with the historical record "Shengnong tried hundreds of herbs and began to set up Chinese medicine".

Preserved in Shanghai Museum of Traditional Chinese Medicine

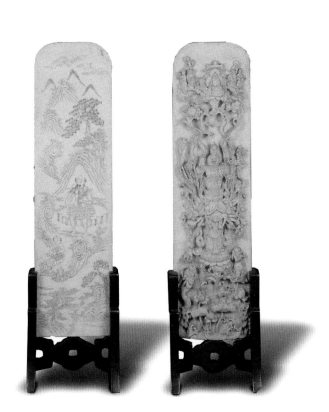

神农尝药牙牌

清

象牙质

宽 8.5 厘米，高 31.5 厘米

左图为正面，右图为背面。

上海中医药博物馆藏

Ivory Domino Carved with Design of Shengnong's Tasting Herb Medicines

Qing Dynasty

Ivory

Width 8.5 cm/ Height 31.5 cm

The picture on the left is the obverse side and the one on the right is the reverse side.

Preserved in Shanghai Museum of Traditional Chinese Medicine

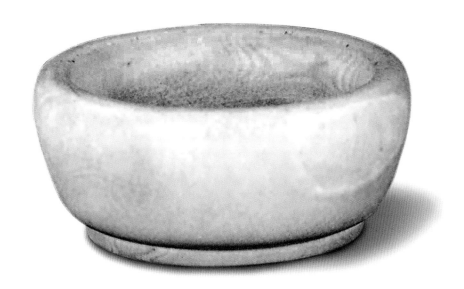

象牙研钵

清

象牙质

口径 8 厘米，高 6.5 厘米

某些药材不宜同铁、铜接触，用此研磨。

上海中医药博物馆藏

Ivory Mortar

Qing Dynasty

Ivory

Mouth Diameter 8 cm/ Height 6.5 cm

The mortar was utilized for porphyrizing some crude drugs which were unsuited in contact with iron and copper.

Preserved in Shanghai Museum of Traditional Chinese Medicine

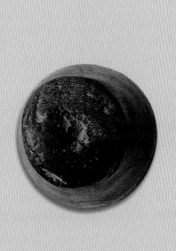
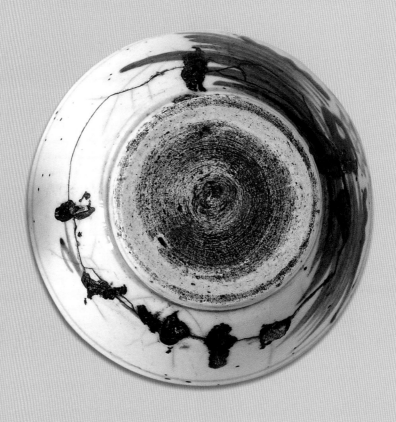

药钵

清

瓷质

口径 15 厘米

这只锔了 8 个铜钉的药钵体现了"没有金刚
钻儿，别揽瓷器活儿"的道理。

上海医药文献博物馆民国馆藏

Medicine Bowl

Qing Dynasty

Porcelain

Mouth Width 15 cm

Mended with 8 cramps, this medicine bowl
has proved the truth of the saying "Without
diamonds, don't do porcelain work."

Preserved in the Museum of Republic of China/
Shanghai Medical Literature Museum

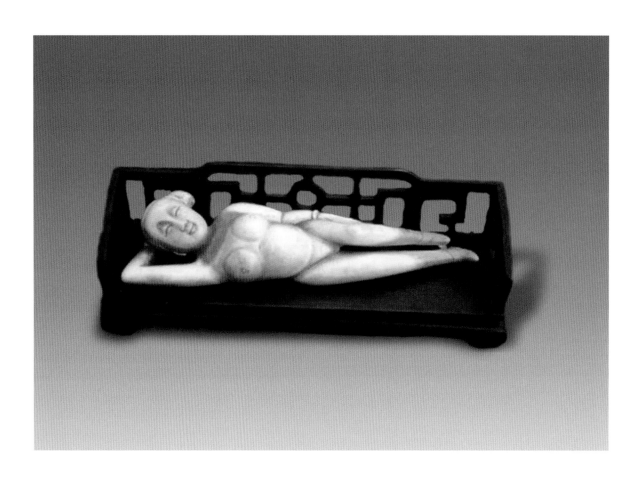

牙雕仕女卧床像

清

象牙质

长 22.2 厘米，重 261 克

Ivory Statue of an Elegant Lady Lying in Bed

Qing Dynasty

Ivory

Length 22.2 cm/ Weight 261 g

在封建社会有"男女授受不亲"的思想，女性生病，医生不能直接检查患者，就在仕女像上告诉医生，患者病痛的部位特征，因此它是医生诊断女性病人的一个道具。

广东中医药博物馆藏

In Chinese feudal society, there used to be an idea and thought that "It was improper for men and women to touch each other's hand in passing objects." So when a female was ill and went to see a doctor, the male doctor should not examine the female patient and give her diagnosis directly. What the patient could do was to tell the doctor the uncomfortable positions of her body and features of the illness by employing this kind of lying in bed statue. Therefore, it was a prop for doctors to give diagnosis to female patients at that time.

Preserved in Guangzhou Chinese Medicine Museum

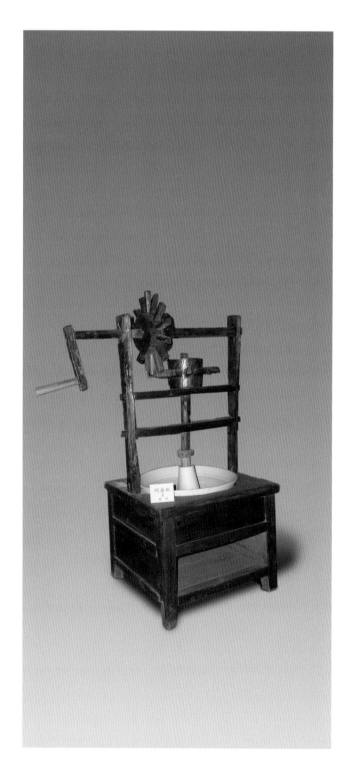

研药机

清

瓷质、木质

研钵：口径 40 厘米，高 12.2 厘米

杵：长 17 厘米

整个研药机：通高 108 厘米

Traditional Chinese Medicine Grinder

Qing Dynasty

Porcelain and Wood

Mortar: Mouth Diameter 40 cm/ Height 12.2 cm

Pestle: 17 cm

Grinder: Height 108 cm

研钵固定于一柜形木架上，并装有木制齿轮传动装置，以备研药省力、方便。制药工具。三级文物，研钵完整，木支架稍残。1983 年入藏。江苏省杨州市同松堂药店征集。

陕西医史博物馆藏

The mortar, equipped with a driving unit of wooden gears, is fixed to a cabinet-shaped wooden support. It was utilized for porphyrizing traditional Chinese medicine. The grinder is energy saving and easy to operate. It was pharmaceutical tool. It is third grade cultural relics. The mortar is in good condition and the wooden support is slightly damaged. It was a collected from the Tong Song Tang Drugstore in Yangzhou of Jiangsu Province, in 1983.

Preserved in Shaanxi Museum of Medicine History

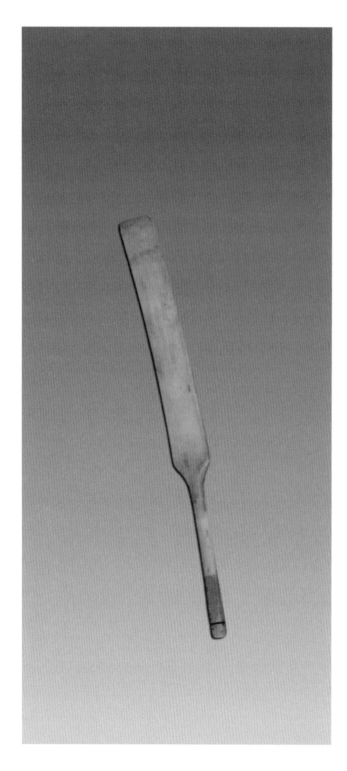

骨药铲

清

骨质

长 12.6 厘米，宽 1.2 厘米，厚 0.4 厘米

Bone Medicine Shovel

Qing Dynasty

Bone

Length 12.6 cm/ Width 1.2 cm/ Thickness 0.4 cm

为动物肢骨片制成。铲形，医用。中医药传统历来讲究药用工具的质地，通常选用骨、角、陶瓷、玻璃和石制品等作材料。这种以动物骨骼制作的药铲在中药的炮制和使用中可以避免药物与工具的化学反应。1954 年入藏，保存完好。

中华医学会／上海中医药大学医史博物馆藏

The shovel is made of the animal's limb bone and was utilized for medical purpose. The traditional Chinese medicine always stresses the material quality of medical tools. Bones, horns, porcelain, glass, and stoneware are always selected as raw material. This kind of medicine shovel can avoid the chemical reaction between medicinal herbs and tools in processing and using Chinese medicine. It was collected in 1954 and is still in good condition.

Preserved in Chinese Medical Association/ Museum of Chinese Medicine, Shanghai University of Traditional Chinese Medicine

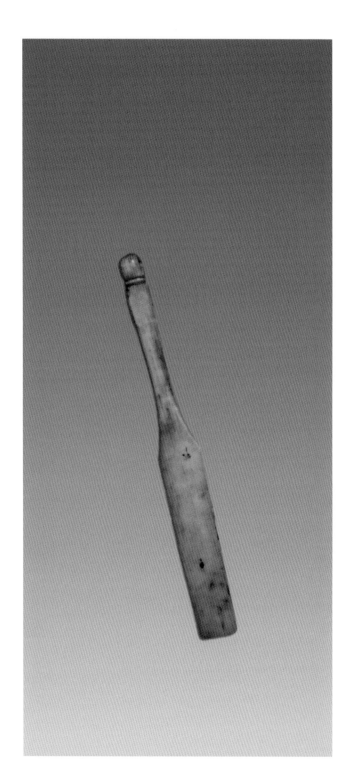

骨药铲

清

骨质

长 8.9 厘米，宽 1.1 厘米，厚 0.5 厘米

Bone Medicine Shovel

Qing Dynasty

Bone

Length 8.9 cm/ Width 1.1 cm/ Thickness 0.5 cm

为动物肢骨片制成。铲形，医用。中医药传统历来讲究药用工具的质地，通常选用骨、角、陶瓷、玻璃和石制品等作材料。这种以动物骨骼制作的药铲在中药的炮制和使用中，可以避免药物与工具的化学反应。1954 年入藏，保存完好。

中华医学会 / 上海中医药大学医史博物馆藏

The shovel is made of the animal's limb bone and was utilized for medical purpose. The traditional Chinese medicine always stresses the material quality of medical tools. Bones, horns, porcelain, glass, and stoneware are always selected as raw material. This kind of medicine shovel can avoid the chemical reaction between medicinal herbs and tools in processing and using Chinese medicine. It was collected in 1954 and is still in good condition.

Preserved in Chinese Medical Association/ Museum of Chinese Medicine, Shanghai University of Traditional Chinese Medicine

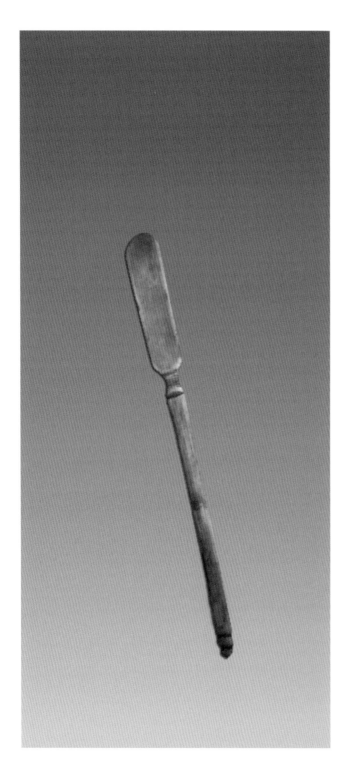

骨药铲

清

骨质

长 12.6 厘米，宽 1.1 厘米，厚 0.3 厘米

Bone Medicine Shovel

Qing Dynasty

Bone

Length 12.6 cm/ Width 1.1 cm/ Thickness 0.3 cm

为动物肢骨片制成。铲形，医用。中医药传统历来讲究药用工具的质地，通常选用骨、角、陶瓷、玻璃和石制品等作材料。这种以动物骨骼制作的药铲在中药的炮制和使用中，可以避免药物与工具的化学反应。1954 年入藏，保存完好。

中华医学会 / 上海中医药大学医史博物馆藏

The shovel is made of the animal's limb bone and was utilized for medical purpose. The traditional Chinese medicine always stresses the material quality of medical tools. Bones, horns, porcelain, glass, and stoneware are always selected as raw material. This kind of medicine shovel can avoid the chemical reaction between medicinal herbs and tools in processing and using Chinese medicine. It was collected in 1954 and is still in good condition.

Preserved in Chinese Medical Association/ Museum of Chinese Medicine, Shanghai University of Traditional Chinese Medicine

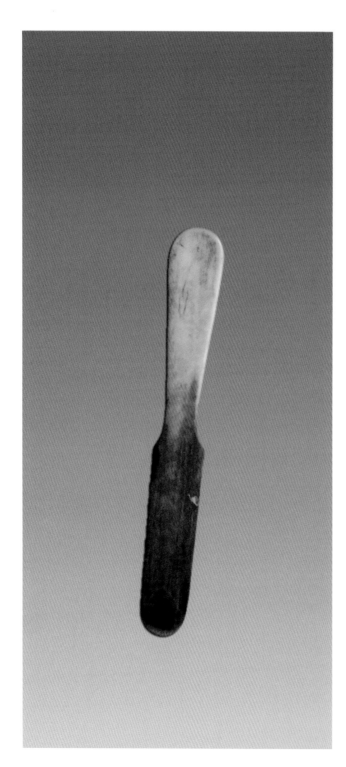

骨药铲

清

骨质

长 18.5 厘米，宽 2.6 厘米，厚 0.6 厘米

Bone Medicine Shovel

Qing Dynasty

Bone

Length 18.5 cm/ Width 2.6 cm/ Thickness 0.6 cm

为动物肢骨片制成。铲形，医用。中医药传统历来讲究药用工具的质地，通常选用骨、角、陶瓷、玻璃和石制品等作材料。这种以动物骨骼制作的药勺在中药的炮制和使用中，可以避免药物与工具的化学反应。1954 年入藏，保存完好。

中华医学会 / 上海中医药大学医史博物馆藏

The shovel is made of the animal's limb bone and was utilized for medical purpose. The traditional Chinese medicine always stresses the material quality of medical tools. Bones, horns, porcelain, glass, and stoneware are always selected as raw material. This kind of medicine shovel can avoid the chemical reaction between medicinal herbs and tools in processing and using Chinese medicine. It was collected in 1954 and is still in good condition.

Preserved in Chinese Medical Association/ Museum of Chinese Medicine, Shanghai University of Traditional Chinese Medicine

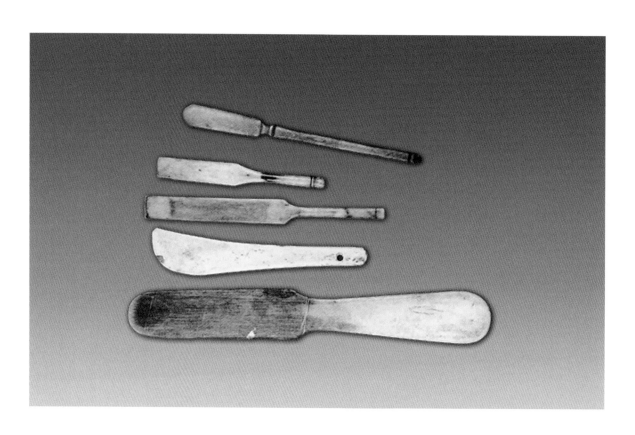

象牙药铲

清

象牙质

调药、量药用具。

上海中医药博物馆藏

Ivory Medicine Shovel

Qing Dynasty

Ivory

The shovel are medical utensils for mixing and measuring medicines.

Preserved in Shanghai Museum of Traditional Chinese Medicine

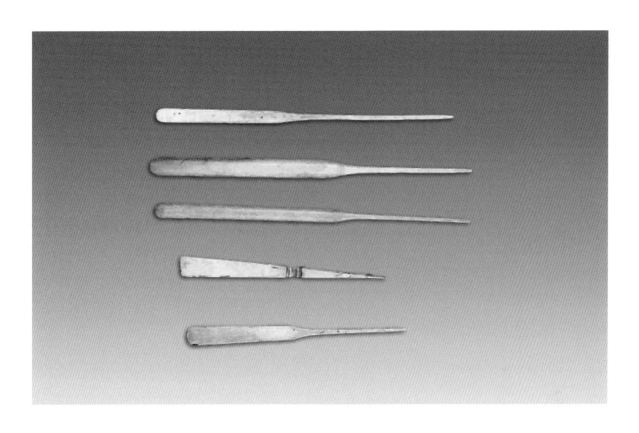

象牙药铲

清

象牙质

调药、量药用具。

上海中医药博物馆藏

Ivory Medicine Shovel

Qing Dynasty

Ivory

The shovel are medical utensils for mixing and measuring medicines.

Preserved in Shanghai Museum of Traditional Chinese Medicine

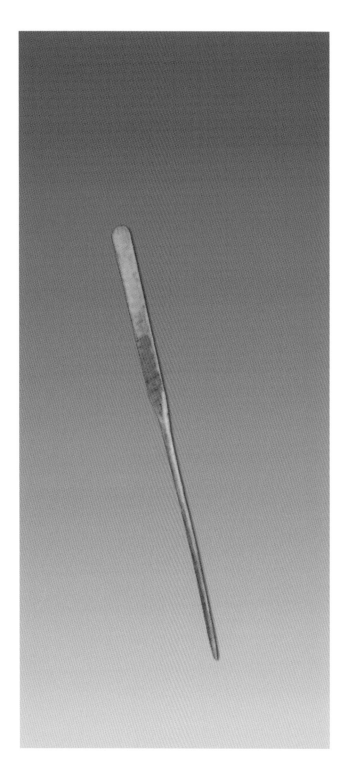

骨药铲

清

骨质

长 15.7 厘米，宽 0.7 厘米，厚 0.2 厘米

Bone Medicine Shovel

Qing Dynasty

Bone

Length 15.7 cm/ Width 0.7 cm/ Thickness 0.2 cm

为动物肢骨片制成。医用。中医药传统历来讲究药用工具的质地,通常选用骨、角、陶瓷、玻璃和石制品等作材料。这种以动物骨骼制作的药勺在中药的炮制和使用中,可以避免药物与工具的化学反应。1954 年入藏,保存完好。

中华医学会 / 上海中医药大学医史博物馆藏

The shovel is made of the animal's limb bone and was utilized for medical purpose. The traditional Chinese medicine always stresses the material quality of medical tools. Bones, horns, porcelain, glass, and stoneware are always selected as raw material. This kind of medicine shovel can avoid the chemical reaction between medicinal herbs and tools in processing and using Chinese medicine. It was collected in 1954 and is still in good condition.

Preserved in Chinese Medical Association/ Museum of Chinese Medicine, Shanghai University of Traditional Chinese Medicine

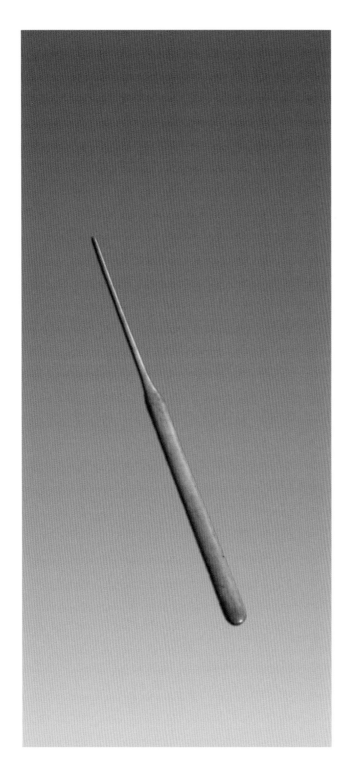

骨药铲

清

骨质

长 16.4 厘米，宽 0.9 厘米，厚 0.3 厘米

Bone Medicine Shovel

Qing Dynasty

Bone

Length 16.4 cm/ Width 0.9 cm/ Thickness 0.3 cm

为动物肢骨片制成。医用。中医药传统历来讲究药用工具的质地，通常选用骨、角、陶瓷、玻璃和石制品等作材料。这种以动物骨骼制作的药勺在中药的炮制和使用中，可以避免药物与工具的化学反应。1954 年入藏，保存完好。

中华医学会 / 上海中医药大学医史博物馆藏

The shovel is made of the animal's limb bone and was utilized for medical purpose. The traditional Chinese medicine always stresses the material quality of medical tools. Bones, horns, porcelain, glass, and stoneware are always selected as raw material. This kind of medicine shovel can avoid the chemical reaction between medicinal herbs and tools in processing and using Chinese medicine. It was collected in 1954 and is still in good condition.

Preserved in Chinese Medical Association/ Museum of Chinese Medicine, Shanghai University of Traditional Chinese Medicine

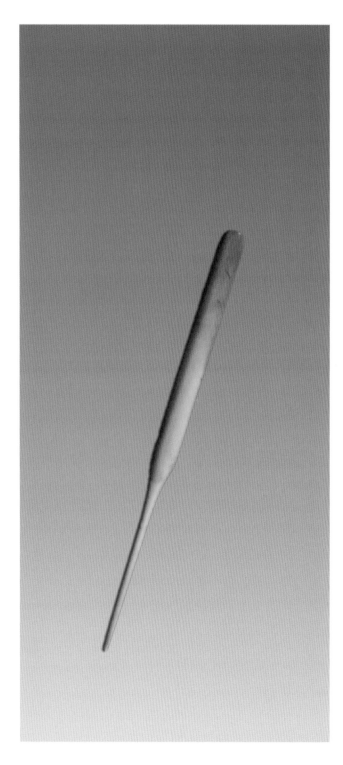

骨药铲

清

骨质

长 16.4 厘米，宽 0.8 厘米，厚 0.2 厘米

Bone Medicine Shovel

Qing Dynasty

Bone

Length 16.4 cm/ Width 0.8 cm/ Thickness 0.2 cm

为动物肢骨片制成。医用。中医药传统历来讲究药用工具的质地，通常选用骨、角、陶瓷、玻璃和石制品等作材料。这种以动物骨骼制作的药勺在中药的炮制和使用中，可以避免药物与工具的化学反应。1954 年入藏，保存完好。

中华医学会 / 上海中医药大学医史博物馆藏

The shovel is made of the animal's limb bone and was utilized for medical purpose. The traditional Chinese medicine always stresses the material quality of medical tools. Bones, horns, porcelain, glass, and stoneware are always selected as raw material. This kind of medicine shovel can avoid the chemical reaction between medicinal herbs and tools in processing and using Chinese medicine. It was collected in 1954 and is still in good condition.

Preserved in Chinese Medical Association/ Museum of Chinese Medicine, Shanghai University of Traditional Chinese Medicine

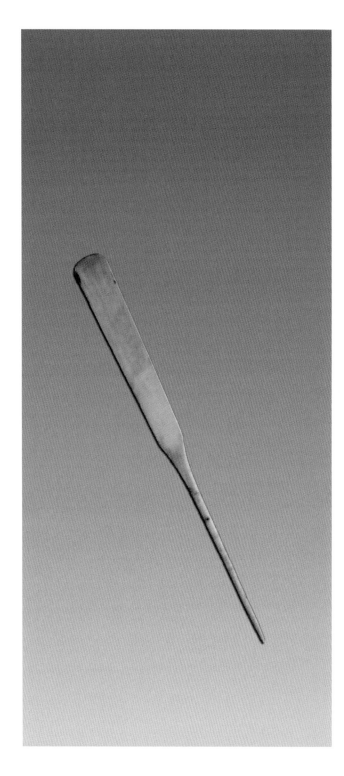

骨药铲

清

骨质

长 11.2 厘米，宽 1 厘米，厚 0.2 厘米

Bone Medicine Shovel

Qing Dynasty

Bone

Length 11.2 cm/ Width 1 cm/ Thickness 0.2 cm

为动物肢骨片制成。医用。中医药传统历来讲究药用工具的质地,通常选用骨、角、陶瓷、玻璃和石制品等作材料。这种以动物骨骼制作的药勺在中药的炮制和使用中,可以避免药物与工具的化学反应。1954 年入藏,保存完好。

中华医学会 / 上海中医药大学医史博物馆藏

The shovel is made of the animal's limb bone and was utilized for medical purpose. The traditional Chinese medicine always stresses the material quality of medical tools. Bones, horns, porcelain, glass, and stoneware are always selected as raw material. This kind of medicine shovel can avoid the chemical reaction between medicinal herbs and tools in processing and using Chinese medicine. It was collected in 1954 and is still in good condition.

Preserved in Chinese Medical Association/ Museum of Chinese Medicine, Shanghai University of Traditional Chinese Medicine

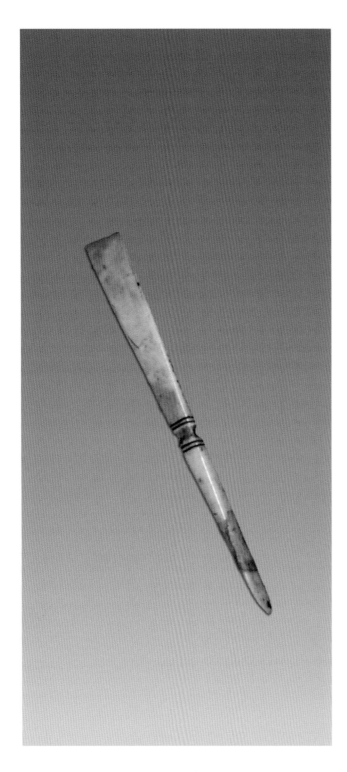

骨药铲

清

骨质

长 10.7 厘米，宽 1 厘米，厚 0.5 厘米

Bone Medicine Shovel

Qing Dynasty

Bone

Length 10.7 cm/ Width 1 cm/ Thickness 0.5 cm

为动物肢骨骨片制成。中医药传统历来讲究药用工具的质地，通常选用骨、角、陶瓷、玻璃和石制品等作材料。这种以动物骨骼制作的药勺在中药的炮制和使用中，可以避免药物与工具的化学反应。1954 年入藏，保存完好。

中华医学会 / 上海中医药大学医史博物馆藏

The shovel is made of the animal's limb bone and was utilized for medical purpose. The traditional Chinese medicine always stresses the material quality of medical tools. Bones, horns, porcelain, glass, and stoneware are always selected as raw material. This kind of medicine shovel can avoid the chemical reaction between medicinal herbs and tools in processing and using Chinese medicine. It was collected in 1954 and is still in good condition.
Preserved in Chinese Medical Association/ Museum of Chinese Medicine, Shanghai University of Traditional Chinese Medicine

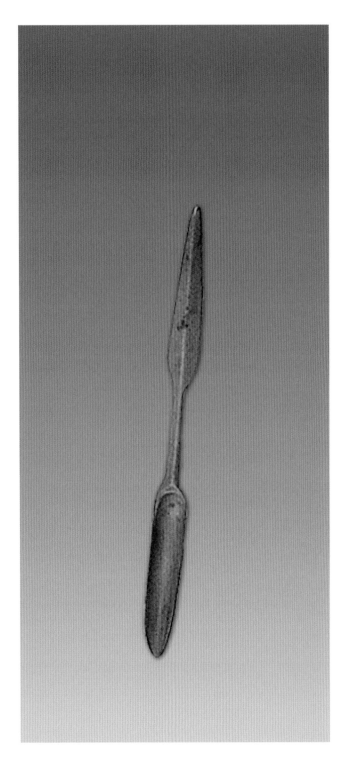

外科药匙

清

木质

通长 17 厘米

匙：长 6.5 厘米，宽 1.2 厘米

柄：长 1.2 厘米

Surgical Medicine Spoon

Qing Dynasty

Wood

Overall Length 17 cm

Spoon: Length 6.5 cm/ Width 1.2 cm

Handle: Length 1.2 cm.

长条形。为外科手术用具。各种形状的大小药匙是外科最常用的上药器具，这是该馆通过自购、征集、受捐等方式收藏展出的 78 件清末中医外科手术用具之一。保存基本完好，匙部有使用痕迹，匙体轻微磨光。

中华医学会 / 上海中医药大学医史博物馆藏

The spoon is in the shape of a long strip. The spoons in various shapes and sizes were most frequently-used tools for applying ointment to the wound in surgery. It was one of the 78 surgical tools utilized during surgical operation in traditional Chinese medicine in the late Qing Dynasty and all of them were collected through purchase, collection, and donation. It is still in good condition with the exception of some used signs of the body and slight wear of the handle. Preserved in Chinese Medical Association/ Museum of Chinese Medicine, Shanghai University of Traditional Chinese Medicine

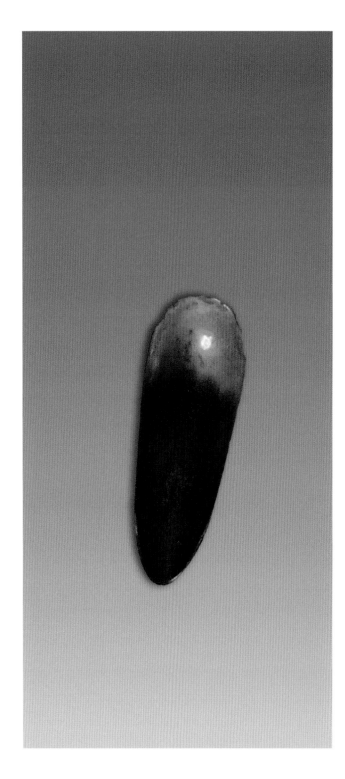

外科药匙

清

牛角质

长 7.9 厘米，宽 2.7 厘米，深 0.9 厘米

Surgical Medicine Scoop

Qing Dynasty

Oxhorn

Length 7.9 cm/ Width 2.7 cm/ Depth 0.9 cm

椭圆形。各种形状大小的药匙是外科最常用
的上药器具，这是该馆通过自购、征集、受
捐等方式收藏展出的78件清末中医外科手
术用具之一。保存基本完好，匙部有使用痕
迹，匙体轻微磨光。

中华医学会/上海中医药大学医史博物馆藏

The spoon is in the shape of oval. The spoons in
various shapes and sizes were most frequently-
used tools for applying ointment to the wound
in surgery. It was one of the 78 surgical tools
utilized for surgical operation in traditional
Chinese medicine in the late Qing Dynasty and
all of them were collected through purchase,
collection, and donation. It is still in good
condition with the exception of some used signs
of the scoop and slight wear of the handle.
Preserved in Chinese Medical Association/
Museum of Chinese Medicine, Shanghai
University of Traditional Chinese Medicine

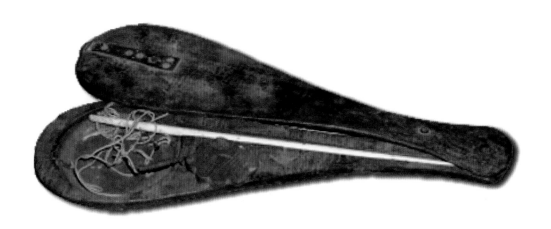

戥子

清

象牙质、铜质

长 29.5 厘米，重 200 克

衡器，完整无损。陕西省礼泉县征集。

陕西医史博物馆藏

Steelyard

Qing Dynasty

Ivory and Bronze

Length 29.5 cm/Weight 200 g

The scale beam of the steelyard is made of ivory, and the scale pan is made of bronze. It was utilized for weighing and is still in good condition. It was collected in Liquan County, Shaanxi Province.

Preserved in Shaanxi Museum of Medicine History

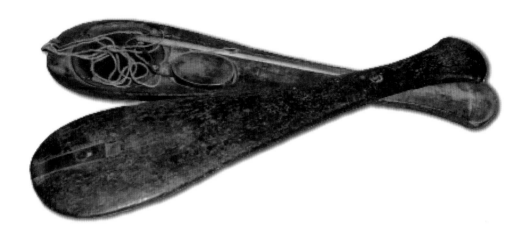

戥子

清

象牙质、铜质

长 36 厘米，重 200 克

衡器，完整无损。陕西省礼泉县征集。

陕西医史博物馆藏

Steelyard

Qing Dynasty

Ivory and Bronze

Length 36 cm/Weight 200 g

The scale beam of the steelyard is made of ivory, and the scale pan is made of bronze. It was utilized for weighing and is still in good condition. It was collected in Liquan County, Shaanxi Province.

Preserved in Shaanxi Museum of Medicine History

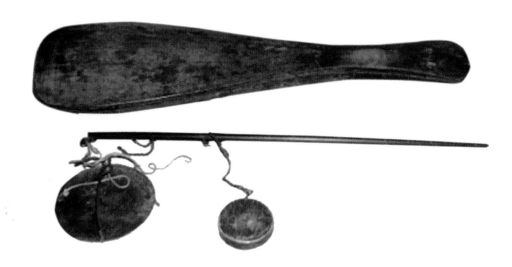

戥子

清

木质、铜质

长35厘米，重200克

衡器，完整无损。陕西省礼泉县征集。

陕西医史博物馆藏

Steelyard

Qing Dynasty

Wood and Bronze

Length 35 cm/Weight 200 g

The scale beam of the steelyard is made of wood, and the scale pan is made of bronze. It was utilized for weighing and is still in good condition. It was collected in Liquan County, Shaanxi Province.

Preserved in Shaanxi Museum of Medicine History

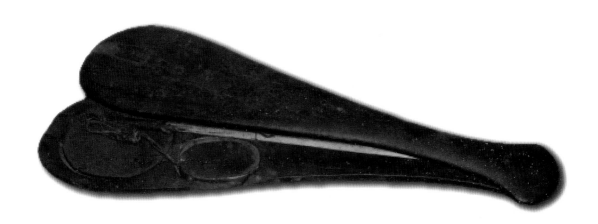

戥子

清

象牙质、铜质

长 35 厘米，重 200 克

衡器，完整无损。陕西省礼泉县征集。

陕西医史博物馆藏

Steelyard

Qing Dynasty

Ivory and Bronze

Length 35 cm/ Weight 200 g

The scale beam of the steelyard is made of ivory, and the scale pan is made of bronze. It was utilized for weighing and is still in good condition. It was collected in Liquan County, Shaanxi Province.

Preserved in Shaanxi Museum of Medicine History

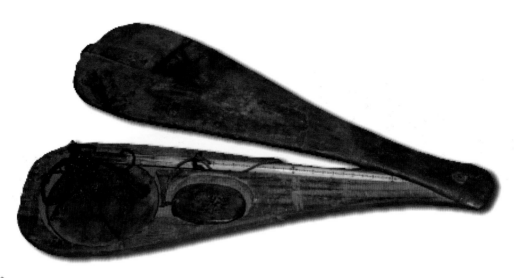

戥子

清

象牙质、铜质

长 32 厘米，重 200 克

衡器，完整无损。陕西省礼泉县征集。

陕西医史博物馆藏

Steelyard

Qing Dynasty

Ivory and Bronze

Length 32 cm/ Weight 200 g

The scale beam of the steelyard is made of ivory, and the scale pan is made of bronze. It was utilized for weighing and is still in good condition. It was collected in Liquan County, Shaanxi Province.

Preserved in Shaanxi Museum of Medicine History

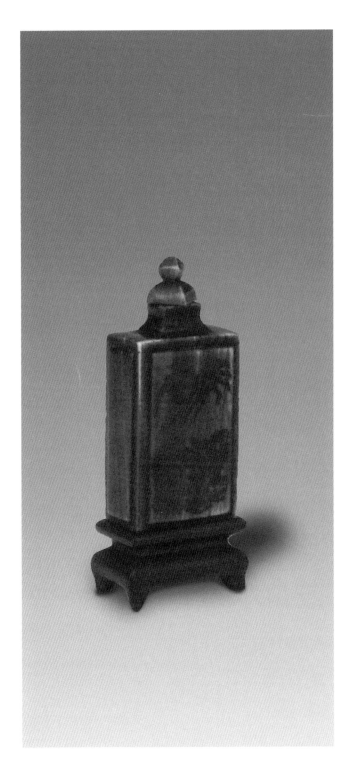

石榴形象牙小药瓶

清

象牙质

底径 4 厘米，高 6 厘米

形似石榴，盖连一小匙，内置药粉。

上海中医药博物馆藏

Pomegranate-shaped Ivory Medicine Bottle

Qing Dynasty

Ivory

Bottom Diameter 4 cm/ Height 6 cm

The bottle is in the shape of a pomegranate with a small spoon on its cap. It was utilized for storing powder medicine.

Preserved in Shanghai Museum of Traditional Chinese Medicine

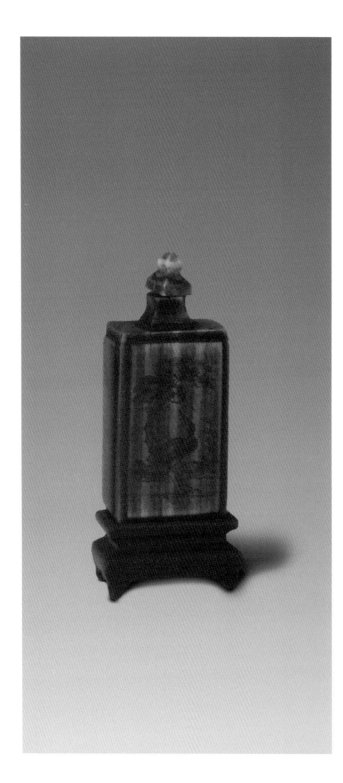

药瓶

清

象牙质

宽 2.6 厘米，厚 1.6 厘米，高 5.7 厘米

Medicine Bottle

Qing Dynasty

Ivory

Width 2.6 cm/ Thickness 1.6 cm/ Height 5.7 cm

扁方状。该瓶褐色，瓶身刻有山水。该瓶用于储存粉末状药物。瓶盖连一小匙，以便存取药粉。1954 年入藏，保存完好。

中华医学会 / 上海中医药大学医史博物馆藏

The bottle is cuboid for storing medicine, It is brown and has a picture of landscape incised on it. especially for storing powdered medicine. A spoon is attached to the cap of the bottle for the convenience of storing and getting medicinal powder. It was collected in 1954 and is still in good condition.

Preserved in Chinese Medical Association/ Museum of Chinese Medicine, Shanghai University of Traditional Chinese Medicine

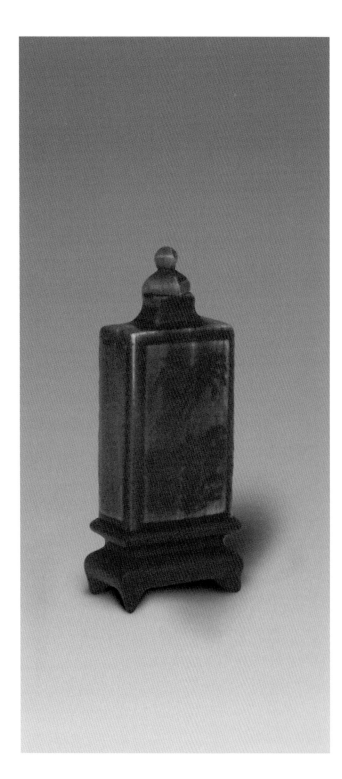

药瓶

清

象牙质

宽 2.6 厘米，厚 1.7 厘米，高 5.7 厘米

Medicine Bottle

Qing Dynasty

Ivory

Width 2.6 cm/ Thickness 1.7 cm/ Height 5.7 cm

扁方状。该瓶褐色，瓶身刻有山水。该藏用
于储存粉末状药物，瓶盖连一小匙，以便存
取药粉。1954 年入藏，保存完好。

中华医学会 / 上海中医药大学医史博物馆藏

The bottle is cuboid for storing medicine,
especially powdered medicine. The bottle is
brown and has a picture of landscape incised on
it. Its cap has a small spoon for the convenience
of storing and getting medicinal powder. It was
collected in 1954 and is still in good condition.
Preserved in Chinese Medical Association/
Museum of Chinese Medicine, Shanghai
University of Traditional Chinese Medicine

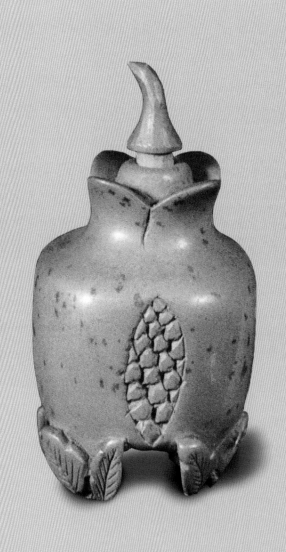

石榴形象牙小药瓶

清

象牙质

底径 4 厘米，高 6 厘米

形似石榴，盖连一小匙，内置药粉。

上海中医药博物馆藏

Pomegranate-shaped Ivory Medicine Bottle

Qing Dynasty

Ivory

Bottom Diameter 4 cm/ Height 6 cm

The bottle is in the shape of a pomegranate with a small spoon on its cap. It was utilized for storing powder medicine.

Preserved in Shanghai Museum of Traditional Chinese Medicine

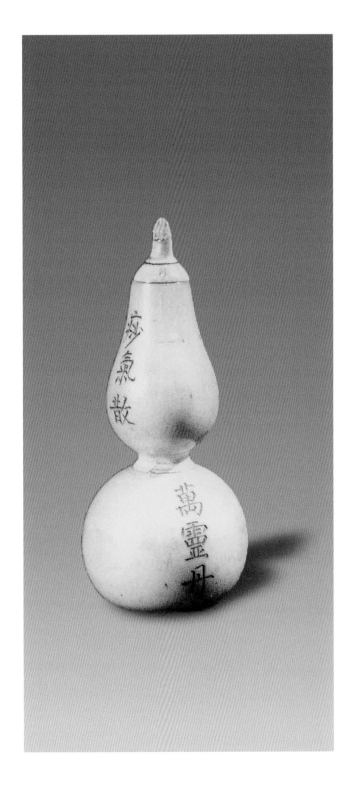

象牙葫芦药瓶

清

象牙质

腹围 9.5 厘米，高 6.5 厘米

Gourd-shaped Ivory Medicine Bottle

Qing Dynasty

Ivory

Belly girth 9.5 cm/ Height 6.5 cm

瓶上刀刻阴书"痧气散""万灵丹"6字。

上海中医药博物馆藏

The bottle is incised with six intaglio Chinese characters "Sha Qi San" and "Wan ling Dan", meaning the names of the drug.

Preserved in Shanghai Museum of Traditional Chinese Medicine

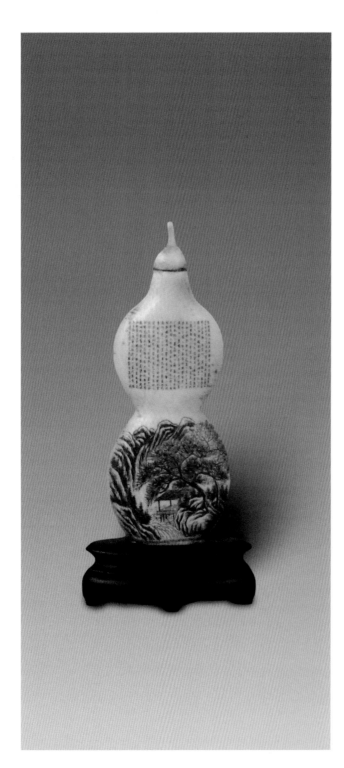

象牙微雕葫芦瓶

清

象牙质

宽3厘米，厚1厘米，通高7厘米

Gourd-shaped Ivory Bottle with Miniature Engraving

Qing Dynasty

Ivory

Width 3 cm/ Thickness 1 cm/ Height 7 cm

扁瓶形。为象牙制成，实心，表面微雕有山水及文字，制作精细，具较高观赏收藏价值。工艺品。1954 年入藏，保存完好。

中华医学会 / 上海中医药大学医史博物馆藏

The ware is in the shape of a flat bottle. The solid ivory bottle was utilized as an artware. Its surface is incised with exquisite miniature landscape and characters. It has high ornamental value for collection. It was collected in 1954 and is still in good condition.

Preserved in Chinese Medical Association/ Museum of Chinese Medicine, Shanghai University of Traditional Chinese Medicine

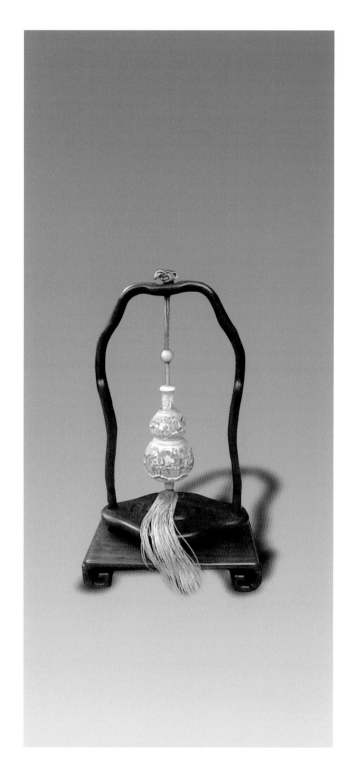

象牙透雕葫芦瓶

清

象牙质

上腹径 4 厘米，下腹径 5.4 厘米，须长

17.2 厘米，通高 9.2 厘米

Gourd-shaped Ivory Bottle Carved in Openwork

Qing Dynasty

Ivory

Upper Belly Diameter 4 cm/ Lower Belly

Diameter 5.4 cm/ Tassel Length 17.2 cm/

Height 9.2 cm

葫芦形，为象牙制成，透雕，表面着色，制作精细，具较高观赏收藏价值。工艺品。1958 年入藏，保存完好。

中华医学会 / 上海中医药大学医史博物馆藏

The ivory bottle is gourd-shaped. It is carved in openwork with surface coloration. It is an exquisite artware of great value for appreciation and collection. It was collected in 1958 and is still in good condition.

Preserved in Chinese Medical Association/ Museum of Chinese Medicine, Shanghai University of Traditional Chinese Medicine

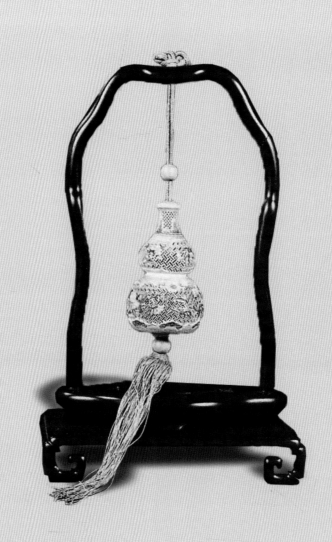

透雕镂空象牙熏瓶

清

象牙质

高 12 厘米

此器全镂空，透雕花卉，填以色彩，制作精美。

上海中医药博物馆藏

Ivory Aroma Bottle Carved in Openwork

Qing Dynasty

Ivory

Height 12 cm

The bottle is carved entirely in openwork which is exquisite with colorful ornamental flowers and plants.

Preserved in Shanghai Museum of Traditional Chinese Medicine

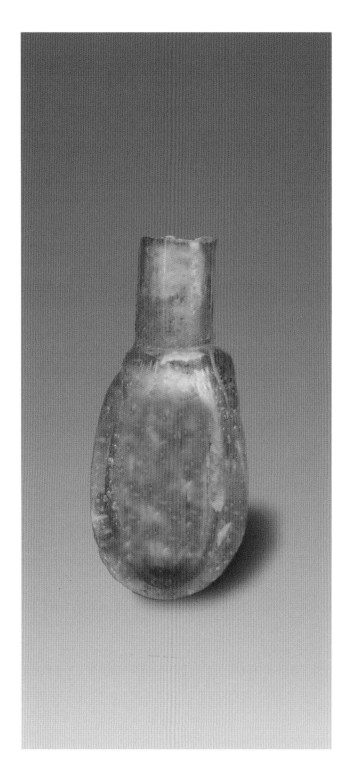

各式小药瓶

清

玻璃质

外口径 0.7 厘米，腹径宽 1.4 厘米，腹径厚
0.9 厘米，通高 3 厘米，重 2 克

玻璃制成，用于装药。

广东中医药博物馆藏

Vial

Qing Dynasty

Glass

Outer Mouth Diameter 0.7 cm/ Belly width
1.4 cm/ Belly thickness 0.9 cm/ Height 3 cm/
Weight 2 g

The bottle is made of glass and for storing
medicines.

Preserved in Guangzhou Chinese Medicine
Museum

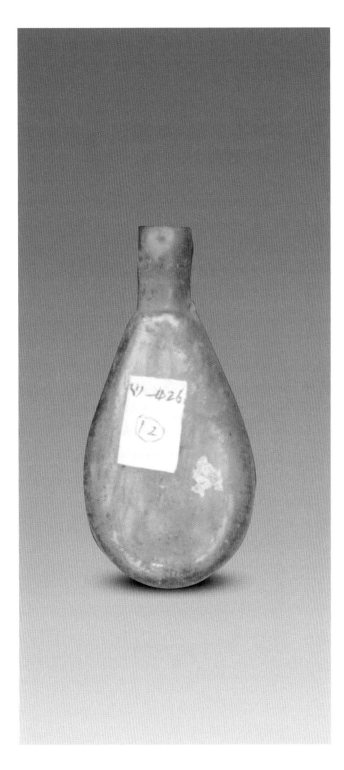

各式小药瓶

清

玻璃质

外口径 1 厘米，径宽 3.3 厘米，腹厚 1.2 厘米，

通高 6.75 厘米，重 13 克

玻璃制成，用于装药。

广东中医药博物馆藏

Vial

Qing Dynasty

Glass

Outer Mouth Diameter 1 cm/ Belly width

3.3 cm/ Belly thickness 1.2 cm/ Height 6.75 cm/

Weight 13 g

The bottle is made of glass and for storing

medicines.

Preserved in Guangzhou Chinese Medicine

Museum

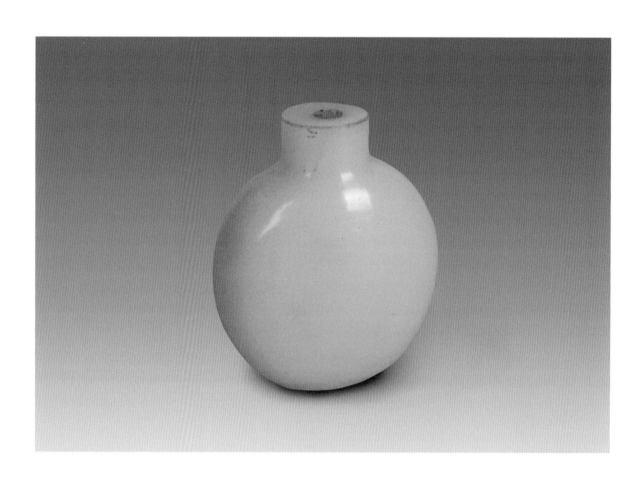

玻璃药瓶

清

玻璃质

口外径 1.65 厘米，口内径 0.54 厘米，宽 4.35 厘米，厚 2.3 厘米，通高 5.1 厘米

Glass Medicine Bottle

Qing Dynasty

Glass

Mouth Outer Diameter 1.65 cm/ Mouth Inner Diameter 0.54 cm/ Width 4.35 cm/ Thickness 2.3 cm/ Height 5.1 cm

扁瓶状。药瓶由乳白色不透明玻璃制成，上口有残。为盛药器具。1955 年入藏，保存基本完好。

中华医学会 / 上海中医药大学医史博物馆藏

The flat bottle is made of milk white opaque glass for storing medicine. It was collected in 1955 and is almost kept intact with only slight damage at its upper mouth.

Preserved in Chinese Medical Association/ Museum of Chinese Medicine, Shanghai University of Traditional Chinese Medicine

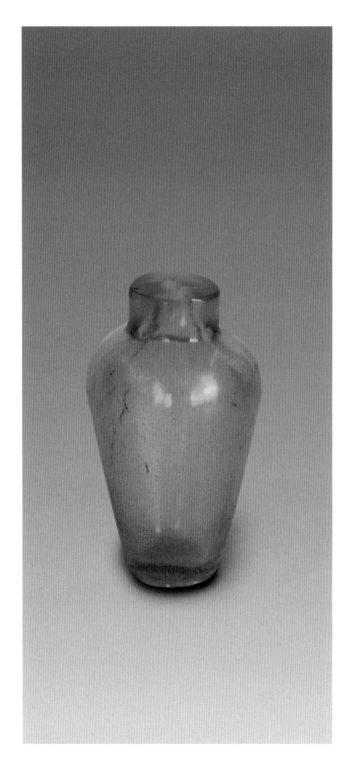

玻璃药瓶

清

玻璃质

腹径 3.12 厘米，通高 5.24 厘米

Glass Medicine Bottle

Qing Dynasty

Glass

Belly Diameter 3.12 cm/ Height 5.24 cm

圆瓶形。药瓶由茶色透明玻璃制成。为盛药器具。1955 年入藏，保存基本完好。

中华医学会 / 上海中医药大学医史博物馆藏

The round bottle is made of tawny transparent glass for storing medicine. It was collected in 1955 and is still in good condition.

Preserved in Chinese Medical Association/ Museum of Chinese Medicine, Shanghai University of Traditional Chinese Medicine

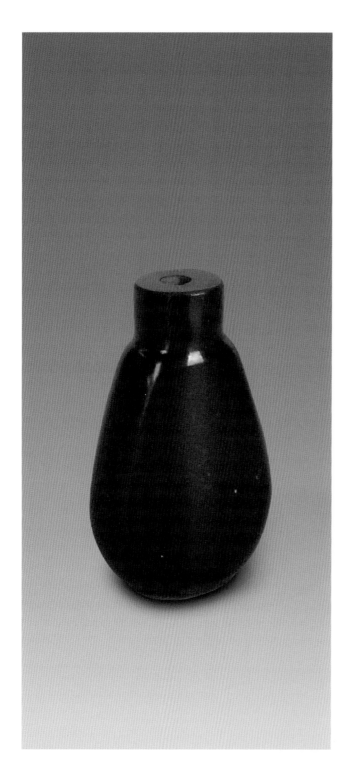

玻璃药瓶

清

玻璃质

宽 3.3 厘米，厚 1.55 厘米，通高 5.95 厘米

Glass Medicine Bottle

Qing Dynasty

Glass

Width 3.3 cm/ Thickness 1.55 cm/ Height 5.95 cm

扁瓶形。药瓶为无色透明玻璃内胎，外有蓝色玻璃饰面，饰面上有文字和竹节图案。为盛药器具。1955 年入藏，保存基本完好。

中华医学会 / 上海中医药大学医史博物馆藏

The flat glass bottle is colorless and transparent and the blue glass wall facing is painted with characters and bamboo-ridge patterns. It was utilized for storing medicine and collected in 1955. It is still in good condition.

Preserved in Chinese Medical Association/ Museum of Chinese Medicine, Shanghai University of Traditional Chinese Medicine

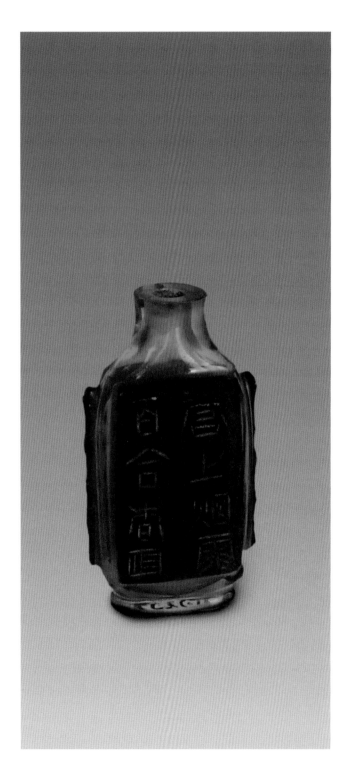

玻璃药瓶

清

玻璃质

宽 3.4 厘米，厚 1.95 厘米，通高 5.45 厘米

Glass Medicine Bottle

Qing Dynasty

Glass

Width 3.4 cm/ Thickness 1.95 cm/ Height 5.45 cm

圆瓶形。药瓶由蓝色不透明玻璃制成。为盛

药器具。1955 年入藏，保存基本完好。

中华医学会 / 上海中医药大学医史博物馆藏

The round bottle is made of blue and black
opaque glass for storing medicine. It was
collected in 1955 and is still in good condition.
Preserved in Chinese Medical Association/
Museum of Chinese Medicine, Shanghai
University of Traditional Chinese Medicine

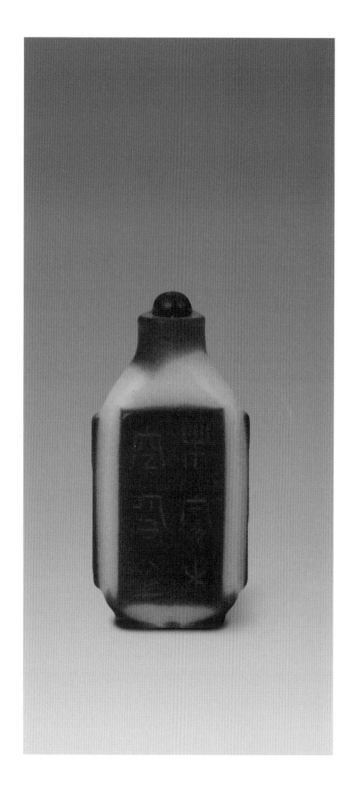

玻璃药瓶

清

玻璃质

口径 1.4 厘米，宽 3.2 厘米，厚 1.6 厘米，

通高 6.6 厘米

Glass Medicine Bottle

Qing Dynasty

Glass

Mouth Diameter 1.4 cm/ Width 3.2 cm/

Thickness 1.6 cm/ Height 6.6 cm

扁瓶形。该藏红白相间，正面红底阴刻"未定木，空殳金"字样，配小红盖，制作精细，造型美观。为盛药器具。1955 年入藏，保存基本完好。

中华医学会 / 上海中医药大学医史博物馆藏

The red and white bottle is flat. The base color of the obverse side is red and is carved in intaglio with the Chinese characters reading "Wei Ding Mu, Kong Shu Jin". The bottle has a red lid and is exquisitely and gracefully shaped. It was utilized for storing medicine. It was collected in 1955 and is still in good conditions. Preserved in Chinese Medical Association/ Museum of Chinese Medicine, Shanghai University of Traditional Chinese Medicine

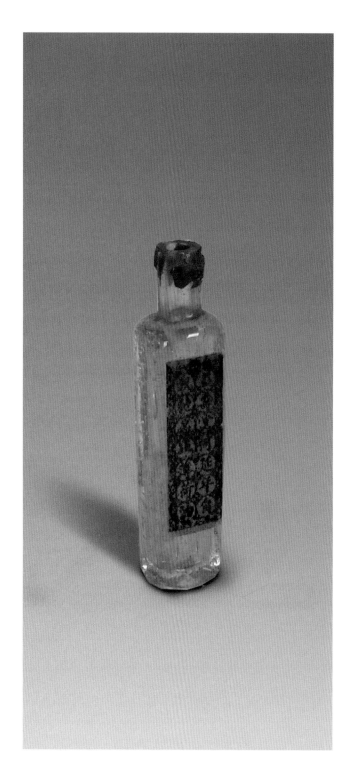

玻璃药瓶

清

玻璃质

宽 1.6 厘米，厚 1.45 厘米，通高 6.7 厘米

Glass Medicine Bottle

Qing Dynasty

Glass

Width 1.6 cm/ Thickness 1.45 cm/ Height 6.7 cm

长方形。药瓶为无色透明玻璃制成，为盛药器具。1955 年入藏，保存基本完好。

中华医学会 / 上海中医药大学医史博物馆藏

The rectangle bottle is made of colorless transparent glass for storing medicine. It was collected in 1955 and is still in good condition.

Preserved in Chinese Medical Association/ Museum of Chinese Medicine, Shanghai University of Traditional Chinese Medicine

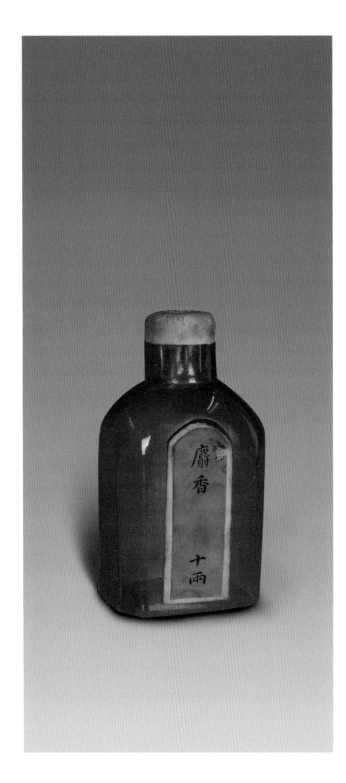

玻璃药瓶

清

玻璃质

宽 9.65 厘米，厚 7.35 厘米，通高 17.2 厘米

Glass Medicine Bottle

Qing Dynasty

Glass

Width 9.65 cm/ Thickness 7.35 cm/ Height 17.2 cm

扁方形。药瓶由无色透明玻璃制成，瓶身一面贴纸标签写有"麝香十两"字样，瓶有玻璃盖。为盛药器具。1986 年入藏，保存基本完好。

中华医学会 / 上海中医药大学医史博物馆藏

The cuboid bottle is made of colorless transparent glass. The bottle has a paper label with the Chinese characters reading "She Xiang Shi Liang" on its one side, meaning the name of the drug. Covered with a glass lid, it was utilized for storing medicine. It was collected in 1986 and is still in good condition.

Preserved in Chinese Medical Association/ Museum of Chinese Medicine, Shanghai University of Traditional Chinese Medicine

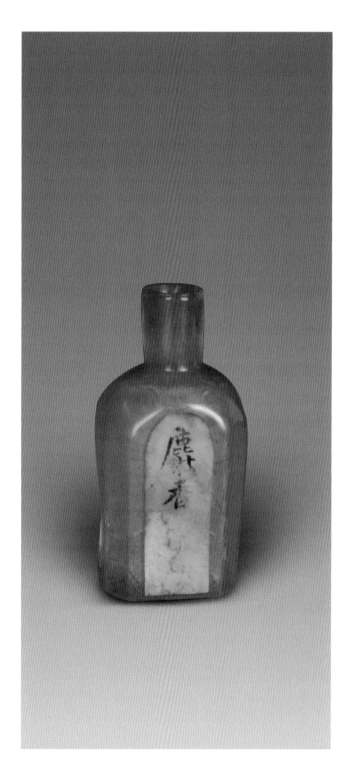

玻璃药瓶

清

玻璃质

宽 5.6 厘米，厚 5.15 厘米，通高 11.3 厘米

Glass Medicine Bottle

Qing Dynasty

Glass

Width 5.6 cm/ Thickness 5.15 cm/ Height 11.3 cm

扁方形。药瓶由无色透明玻璃制成，瓶身一

面贴纸标签写有"麝香"字样。为盛药器具。

1986 年入藏，有多处裂痕。

中华医学会 / 上海中医药大学医史博物馆藏

The cuboid bottle is made of colorless transparent glass for storing medicine. The bottle has a paper label with the Chinese characters reading "She Xiang" on its one side, meaning the name of the drug. The bottle was collected in 1986. It has many cracks.

Preserved in Chinese Medical Association/ Museum of Chinese Medicine, Shanghai University of Traditional Chinese Medicine

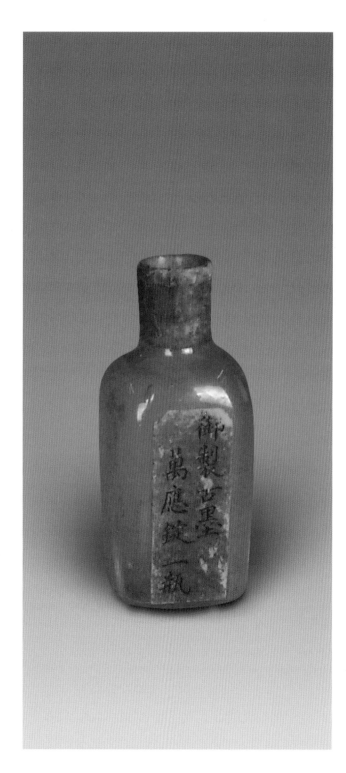

玻璃药瓶

清

玻璃质

宽 2.6 厘米，厚 2.5 厘米，通高 6.05 厘米

Glass Medicine Bottle

Qing Dynasty

Glass

Width 2.6 cm/ Thickness 2.5 cm/ Height 6.05 cm

扁方形。药瓶由无色透明玻璃制成，瓶身一面贴纸标签写有"御制古墨万应锭一瓶"字样。为盛药器具。故宫博物院捐赠。1986 年入藏，保存基本完好。

中华医学会 / 上海中医药大学医史博物馆藏

The cuboid bottle is made of colorless transparent glass for storing medicine. The bottle has a paper label with the Chinese characters reading "Yu Zhi Gu Mo Wan Ying Ding Yi Ping" on its one side, meaning the name of the drug. It was collected in 1986 and is still in good condition.

Preserved in Chinese Medical Association/ Museum of Chinese Medicine, Shanghai University of Traditional Chinese Medicine

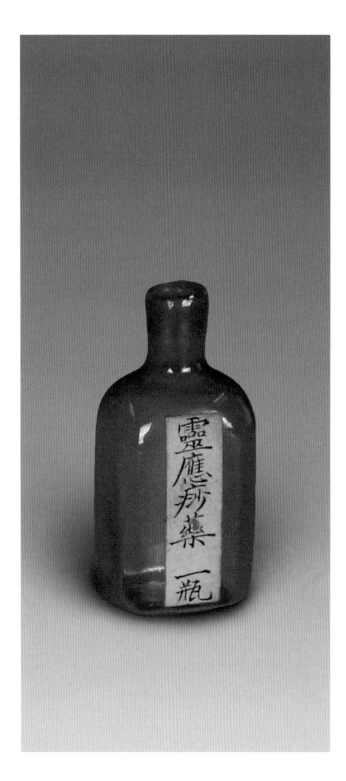

玻璃药瓶

清

玻璃质

宽 2.65 厘米，厚 2.45 厘米，通高 5.5 厘米

Glass Medicine Bottle

Qing Dynasty

Glass

Width 2.65 cm/ Thickness 2.45 cm/ Height 5.5 cm

扁方形。药瓶由无色透明玻璃制成，瓶身一面贴纸标签写有"灵应痧药一瓶"字样。为盛药器具。故宫博物院捐赠。1986 年入藏，保存基本完好。

中华医学会 / 上海中医药大学医史博物馆藏

The cuboid bottle is made of colorless transparent glass for storing medicine. The bottle has a paper label with the Chinese characters reading "Ling Ying Sha Yao Yi Ping" on its one side, meaning the name of the drug. It was collected in 1986 and is still in good condition.

Preserved in Chinese Medical Association/ Museum of Chinese Medicine, Shanghai University of Traditional Chinese Medicine

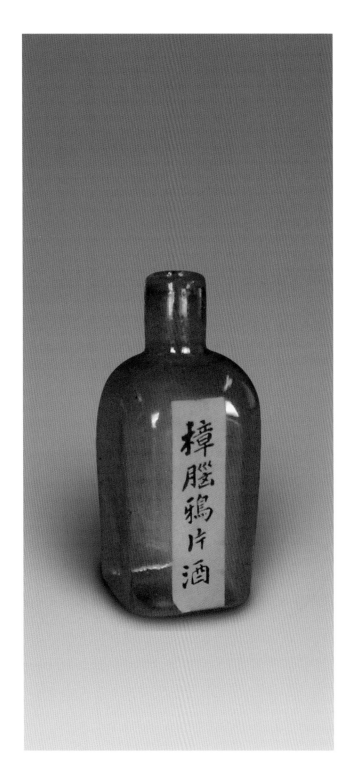

玻璃药瓶

清

玻璃质

宽 4 厘米，厚 4 厘米，通高 8.65 厘米

Glass Medicine Bottle

Qing Dynasty

Glass

Width 4 cm/ Thickness 4 cm/ Height 8.65 cm

扁方形。药瓶由无色透明玻璃制成，瓶身一
面贴纸标签写有"樟脑鸦片酒"字样。为盛
药器具。1986 年入藏。保存基本完好。

中华医学会 / 上海中医药大学医史博物馆藏

The cuboid bottle is made of colorless transparent
glass for storing medicine. The bottle has a paper
label with the Chinese characters reading "Zhang
Nao Ya Pian Jiu" on its one side, meaning the
name of the drug. It was collected in 1986 and is
still in good condition.

Preserved in Chinese Medical Association/
Museum of Chinese Medicine, Shanghai
University of Traditional Chinese Medicine

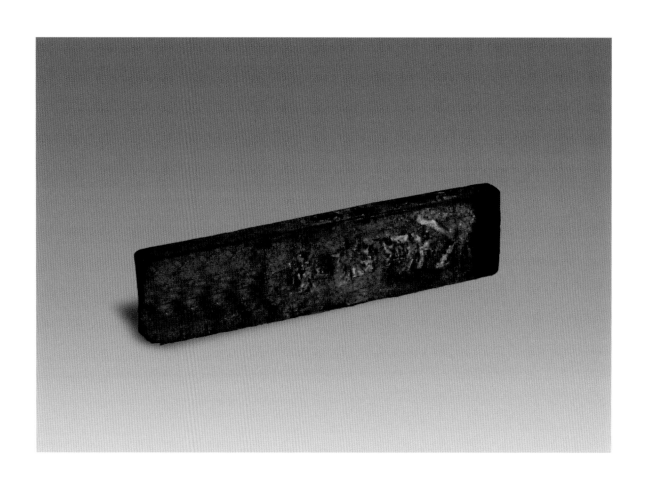

八宝药墨

清

墨质

长 8.4 厘米，高 2 厘米，厚 0.8 厘米

Babao Yaomo Troche

Qing Dynasty

Pine-Soot Ink

Length 8.4 cm/ Height 2 cm/ Thickness 0.8 cm

方柱形。该藏为四面皆有字，分别刻"八宝药墨""药印川□""康熙乙酉"等字样。墨质一般，表面一端有水渍和小裂纹。为文房用品。1964 年入藏。

中华医学会 / 上海中医药大学医史博物馆藏

The collection is square and engraved with Chinese characters on all sides, such as "Ba Bao Yao Mo", "Yao Yin Chuang Kou" and "Kang Xi Yi You". The quality of the ink is ordinary. There is water mark and small cracks at one end of the troche surface. It was an article for use in study and was collected in 1964.

Preserved in Chinese Medical Association/ Museum of Chinese Medicine, Shanghai University of Traditional Chinese Medicine

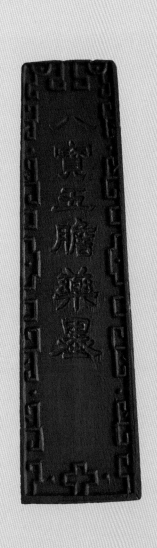

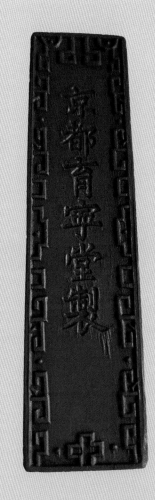

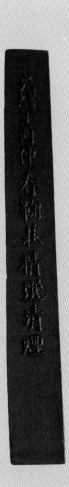

八宝五胆药墨

清

墨质

长 8 厘米，厚 1 厘米

红色，正面刻有"八宝五胆药墨"，背面刻有"京都育宁堂制"。侧面刻有"光绪丁酉仲春鞠庄精选清烟"。药之入墨，古已有之。南唐时期徽墨已名噪全国，药墨随之问世。史载：清光绪年间，八国联军入侵京城，慈禧西逃途中罹患背疮（鱼鳞病）顽疾，寻遍诸药不治，得"八宝五胆药墨"而愈。

新昌县天姥中医博物馆藏

Babao Wudan Cinnabar Stick (Medicinal Ink)

Qing Dynasty

Pine-Soot Ink

Length 8 cm/ Height 1 cm

The collection has a red body part with "Ba Bao Wu Dan Yao Mo" carved on the front and "Jing Du Yu Ning Tang Zhi " on the back. The side is engraved with "Guang Xu Ding You Zhong Chun Ju Zhuang Jing Xuan Qing Yan". The practice to mix medicine in the ink sticks appeared very early. During the Southern Tang Dynasty, ink sticks produced in Huizhou, Anhui were well known all over the country, and medicine ink sticks were created ever since. It was recorded in history that in Guangxu Period, Qing dynasty, the Eight-power Allied Forces invaded into Beijing and Empress Dowager Cixi fled westward to Xi'an and on her way she suffered from back sore (ichthyosis). Many medicines were used but ineffective and only "BabaoWudan Cinnabar Stick" worked.

Preserved in Tianmu Traditional Chinese Medicine Museum of Xinchang County

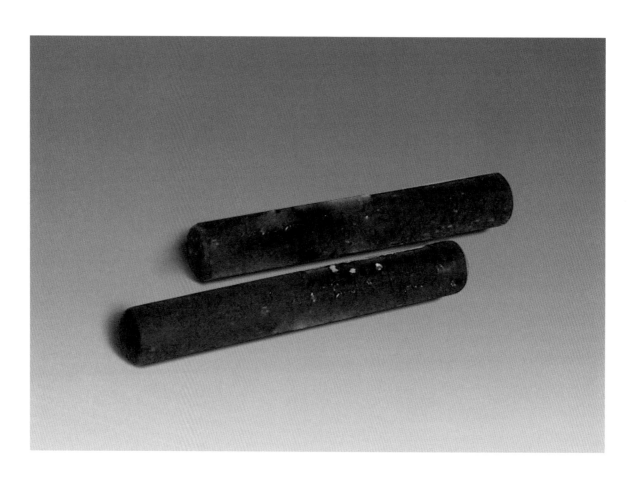

虔制药墨

清

墨质

直径 10 厘米，通长 72 厘米

Qianzhi Yaomo

Qing Dynasty

Pine-Soot Ink

Diameter 10 cm/ Length 7.2 cm

圆柱形。该藏表面刻"徽歙曹德酬孙云崖民监造""虔制药墨"字样，墨头一端刻"素功"两字。为文房用品。1964 年入藏。

中华医学会 / 上海中医药大学医史博物馆藏

The ink is cylindrical. The surface of the ink is engraved with the Chinese characters "Hui Xi Cao De Chou Sun Yun Ya Min Jian Zao" and "Qian Zhi Yao Mo", meaning the name of the manufacturer and the brand respectively. Two characters "Su Gong" are engraved at the head end of the ink pastille. It was an article for use in study and was collected in 1964.

Preserved in Chinese Medical Association/ Museum of Chinese Medicine, Shanghai University of Traditional Chinese Medicine

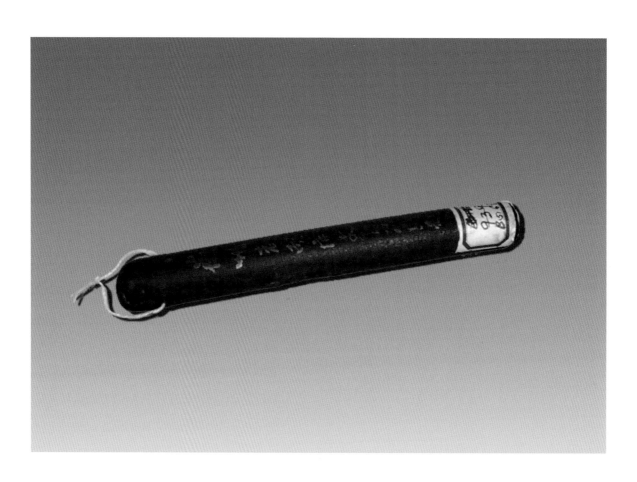

徽州老胡开文松烟圆柱墨

清

墨质

直径 2.1 厘米，通长 19.2 厘米

Cylinder-shaped Pine-soot Ink made by Hu Kaiwen from Huizhou

Qing dynast

Pine-Soot Ink

Diameter 2.1 cm/ Length 19.2 cm

圆柱形。该藏为徽州松烟墨，墨质细腻凝重，表面较圆润光滑。柱身落款模糊不清。为文房用品。1991 年入藏。

中华医学会 / 上海中医药大学医史博物馆藏

The cylinder-shaped collection is Pine-soot Ink from Huizhou. The ink is exquisite, smooth and thick. Its surface is mellow, full and glossy. The inscriptions on the ink pastille are blurred and indistinct. It was an article for use in study and was collected in 1991.

Preserved in Chinese Medical Association/ Museum of Chinese Medicine, Shanghai University of Traditional Chinese Medicine

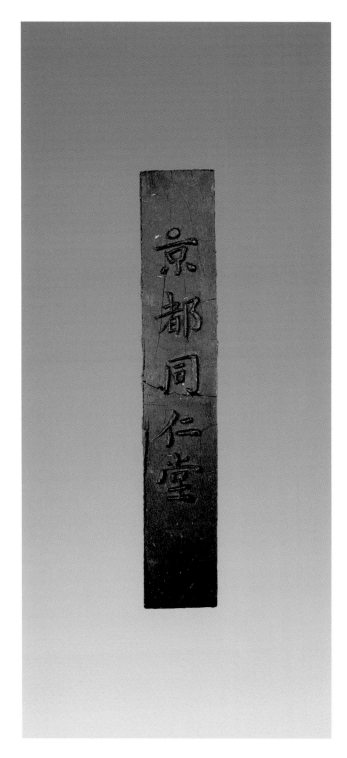

京都同仁堂药墨

清

墨质

长 8.5 厘米，宽 1.7 厘米

Beijing Tong Ren Tang Yaomo

Qing Dynasty

Pine-Soot Ink

Length 8.5 cm/ Width 1.7 cm

康熙乙酉年间的药墨。上有"店堂"及"纪年"双款识。

张雅宗藏

The medicine ink stick was made in Kangxi Yiyou Year (1705), with the name of the shop and manufacturing time engraved on the body part.

Collected by Zhang Yazong

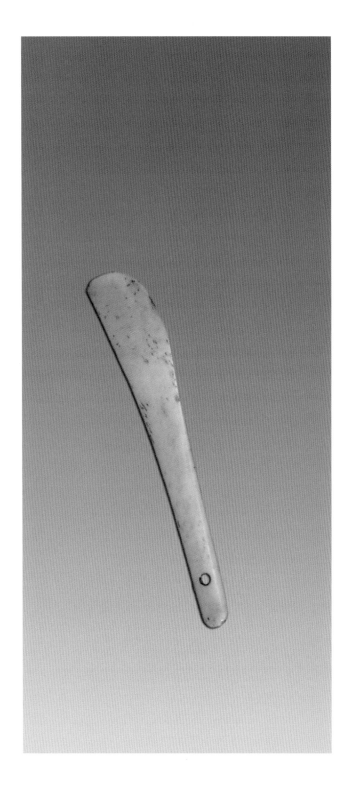

骨刀

清

骨质

长 11.3 厘米，宽 2 厘米，厚 0.5 厘米

Bone Knife

Qing Dynasty

Bone

Length 11.3 cm/ Width 2 cm/ Thickness 0.5 cm

刀形，为动物肢骨骨片制成。医用，用于外科。

1959 年入藏，保存完好。

中华医学会 / 上海中医药大学医史博物馆藏

Shaped as a knife, it is made of the animal's limb bone. It was utilized for medical purpose, especially for surgery. It was collected in 1959 and is still in good condition.

Preserved in Chinese Medical Association/ Museum of Chinese Medicine, Shanghai University of Traditional Chinese Medicine

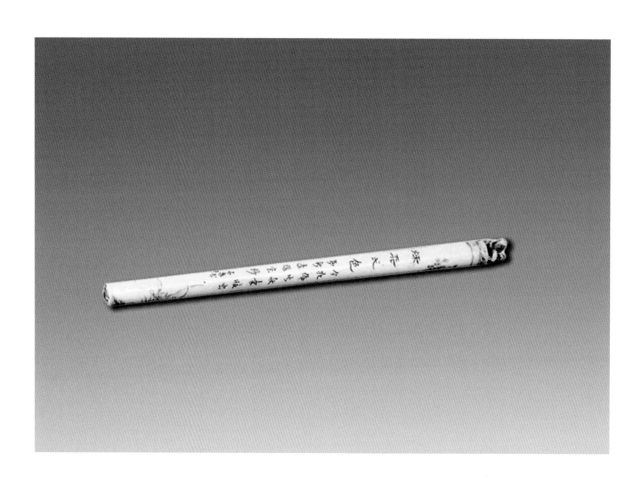

象牙藏针筒

清

象牙质

口径 1.2 厘米，长 22.5 厘米

Ivory Needle Container

Qing Dynasty

Ivory

Mouth Diameter 1.2 cm/ Length 22.5 cm

盖上饰以虎钮。正面刻有隶书"秋天一色",

背面刻有兰花、梅花纹饰。

上海中医药博物馆藏

The cap of the container is decorated with a tiger-shaped knob. The obverse side of the container is engraved with official scripts "Qiu Tian Yi Se", meaning in autumn all plants have the same color, and the reverse side is decorated with the engraved patterns of orchid and plum blossom.

Preserved in Shanghai Museum of Traditional Chinese Medicine

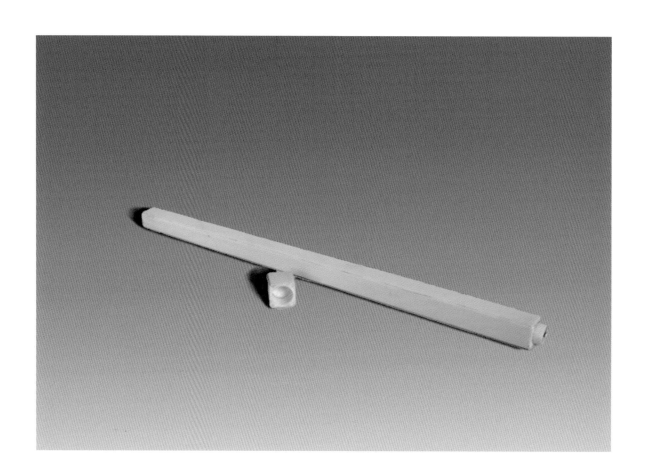

象牙藏针筒

清

象牙质

长 24.3 厘米，宽 1.2 厘米

Ivory Needle Container

Qing Dynasty

Ivory

Length 24.3 cm/ Width 1.2 cm

方柱形，为象牙制品。用于放置针灸用针。

1956 年入藏，保存完好，有使用痕迹。

中华医学会 / 上海中医药大学医史博物馆藏

The container is in the shape of a square column and is an ivory product. It was utilized for storing acupuncture needles. It was collected in 1956 and is still in good condition with the exception of some used traces.

Preserved in Chinese Medical Association/ Museum of Chinese Medicine, Shanghai University of Traditional Chinese Medicine

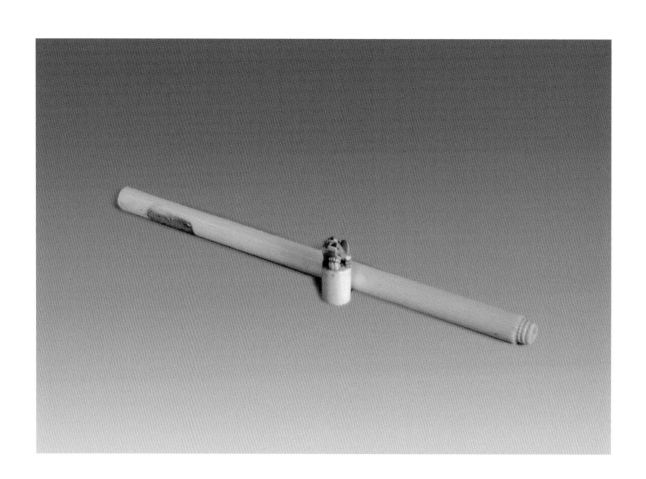

象牙藏针筒

清

象牙质

筒外径 1.05 厘米，内径 0.53 厘米，通长 21.6 厘米

Ivory Needle Container

Qing Dynasty

Ivory

Outer Diameter 1.05 cm/ Inner Diameter 0.53 cm/ Length 21.6 cm

圆管形。为象牙制品，带螺旋纹口盖，盖顶
刻有兽钮。用于放置针灸用针。1954 年入藏，
保存完好，有使用痕迹。

中华医学会 / 上海中医药大学医史博物馆藏

The container is in the shape of a circular tube
and is an ivory product. It was utilized for
storing acupuncture needles. Its spiral cap is
engraved with animal button design. It was
collected in 1954 and is still in good condition
with the exception of some used traces.
Preserved in Chinese Medical Association/
Museum of Chinese Medicine, Shanghai
University of Traditional Chinese Medicine

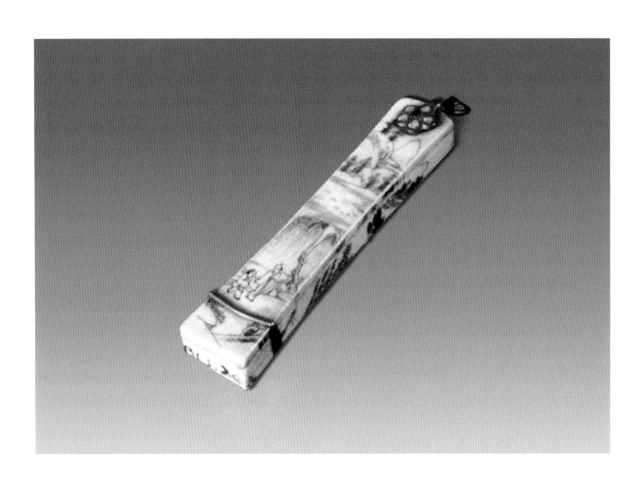

象牙针盒

清

象牙质

长 10 厘米，宽 2 厘米，高 1.5 厘米

Ivory Needle Case

Qing Dynasty

Ivory

Length 10 cm/ Width 2 cm/ Height 1.5 cm

外周阴刻山水人物图，填以墨色。

上海中医药博物馆藏

The case is intaglioed with the patterns of
landscape and figures and painted with ink
color.
Preserved in Shanghai Museum of Traditional
Chinese Medicine

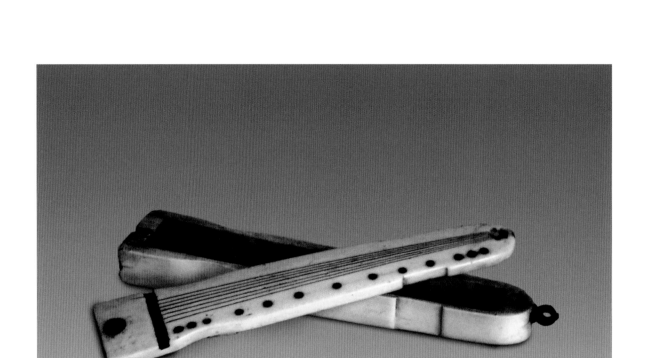

象牙藏针盒

清

象牙质

通长 10.65 厘米，宽 2.1 厘米，厚 1.5 厘米

Ivory Needle Case

Qing Dynasty

Ivory

Length 10.65 cm/ Width 2.1 cm/ Thickness 1.5 cm

古琴形。盒盖刻有琴弦，盒底刻"窗下短檠燃夜雨，塞边长剑倚秋风"，落款"领山书"，详情待考。该藏用于放置针灸用针。1959 年入藏，保存完好，有使用痕迹。

中华医学会 / 上海中医药大学医史博物馆藏

The case is in the shape of a guqin. It was utilized for storing acupuncture needles. The case cover is carved with the pattern of music wires, and the bottom is incised with a rhyming couplet"Chuang Xia Duan Qing Ran Ye Yu, Sai Bian Chang Jian Yi Qiu Feng". An inscription of "Ling Shan Shu"is at the end of the couplet, which might be the craftsman's name but still need to be verified. It was collected in 1959 and is still in good condition with the exception of some used traces.

Preserved in Chinese Medical Association/ Museum of Chinese Medicine, Shanghai University of Traditional Chinese Medicine

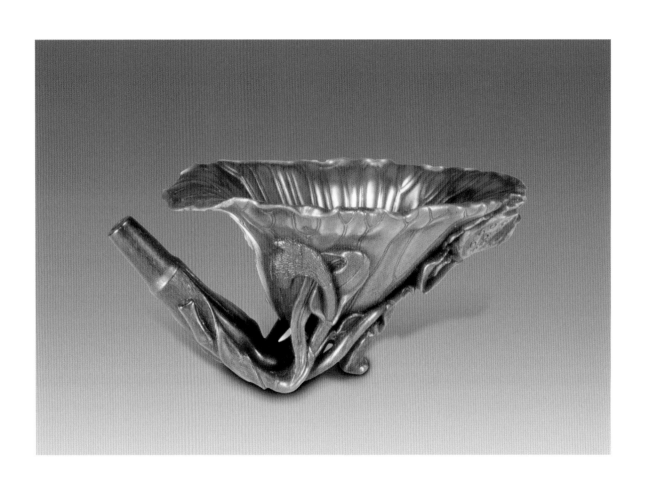

犀角雕莲蓬荷叶杯

清

犀角质

口长径 16.8 厘米，口短径 10.6 厘米，高 16 厘米

Rhinoceros Horn Cup Carved with Lotus Seedpods and Leaves

Qing Dynasty

Rhinoceros Horn

Mouth Long Diameter 16.8 cm/ Mouth Short Diameter 10.6 cm/ Height 16 cm

广角制。匠人以束花莲叶为题材，将长形犀角加工成荷叶杯，流口内弯上翘，杯口敞阔外撇如荷叶形状，荷叶根根筋脉遒劲浅显。杯下镂刻莲花盛开，花蕊结莲蓬，点衬微卷小荷叶。1985 年，香港著名医生叶义捐献。

故宫博物院藏

The cup is made of rhinoceros horn. The craftsman carved the long horn into a lotus-shaped cup based in the form of bunches of flowers and lotus leaves. The head part curves inward and is tip-tilted. The rim of the cup is open wide and flared like a lotus leaf. The ribs of the lotus root are vigorous and obvious. Enchased lotus flowers are blooming at the bottom. With flower pistil knotting the seedpod, lotus seeds are growing in the center. The collection was donated in 1985 by Mr. Ye Yi, a famous Hong Kong doctor.

Preserved in The Palace Museum

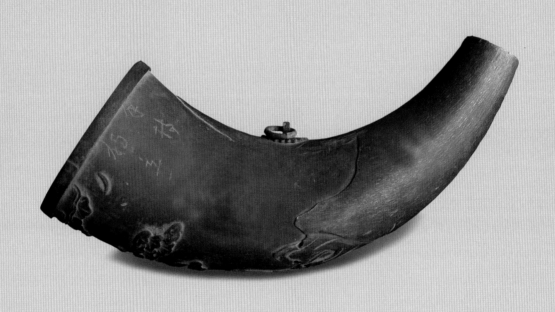

角筒

清

犀角质

小口径 10.5 厘米，大口径 14.5 厘米，长 15 厘米

清代医家尹小泉用品。有人认为是随身盛药用。

江苏省中医药博物馆藏

Horn-shaped Canister

Qing Dynasty

Rhinoceros Horn

Small Mouth Diameter 10.5 cm/ Large Mouth
Diameter 14.5 cm/Length 15 cm

The canister belonged to Yi Xiaoquan, a doctor in
Qing Dynasty. It was considered as a container of
medicine for personal use.

Jiangsu Museum of Traditional Chinese Medicine

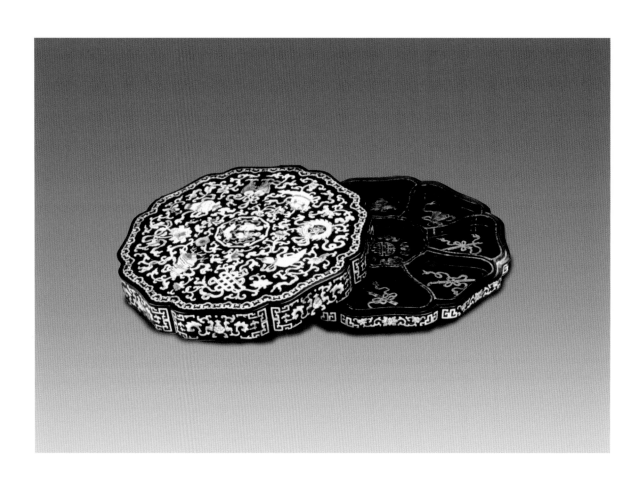

螺钿食盒

清

木质

直径 39 厘米，高 8.5 厘米

Mother-of-pearl Inlay Hamper

Qing Dynasty

Wood

Diameter 39 cm/ Height 8.5 cm

盒呈荷叶形，黑漆地，子母口，四只矮足。
通体由彩色螺钿镶嵌。

山西博物院藏

The hamper is shaped as a lotus leaf with black
lacquer as its background. The hamper has
four short feet and two matching mouths that
seal the cover tightly. The whole wood body is
inlaid with colorful mother-of-pearl.

Preserved in Shanxi Museum

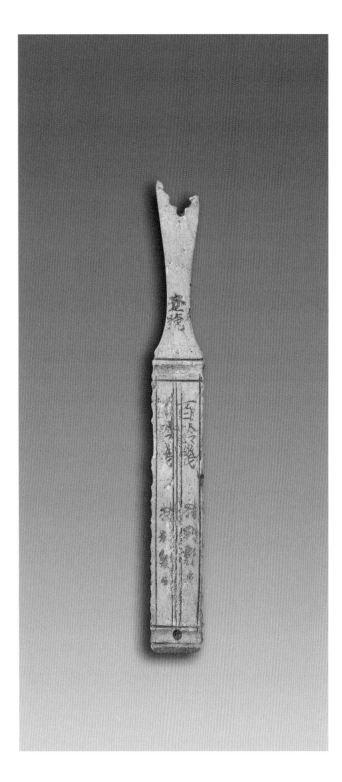

骨酒令

清

骨质

宽 1.1 厘米，高 8 厘米

Bone Token of Drinkers' Wager Game

Qing Dynasty

Bone

Width 1.1 cm/ Height 8 cm

呈象牙黄色。柄部有编号，令身刻铭辞。制作较为简朴。南京大行宫小学出土。

中山陵园管理局藏

The collection is ivory yellow. A serial number is carved on the handle and the inscriptions are incised on the body. The whole token is simple in making. It was unearthed in Daxinggong Primary School in Nanjing.

Preserved in Sun Yatsen Mausoleum Park

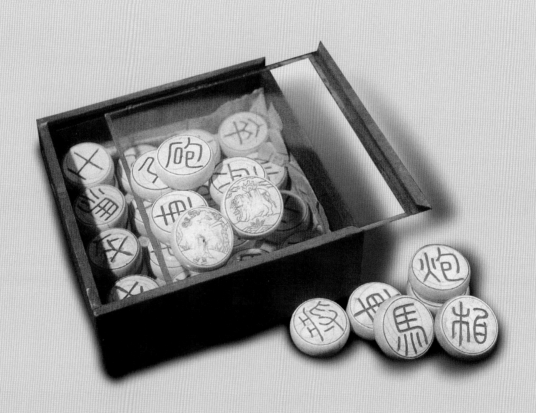

象棋

清

象牙质

象棋子直径 3.5 厘米，厚 2 厘米

象棋子为象牙磨制，一面刻棋子名，另一面刻相应的图案，共计 32 颗。其中阴刻篆书填红 16 颗，阴刻篆书填墨 16 颗。皆盛在一长方形木盒内。

中国体育博物馆藏

Chinese Chess

Qing Dynasty

Ivory

Piece diameter 3.5 cm/ Thickness 2 cm

The chess pieces, with name on one side and corresponding patterns on the other side, are grinded and polished from ivory. There are 32 pieces in total, half of which are carved in red seal character in intaglio and the other half in black. All the pieces are stored in a rectangular wooden box.

Preserved in China Sports Museum

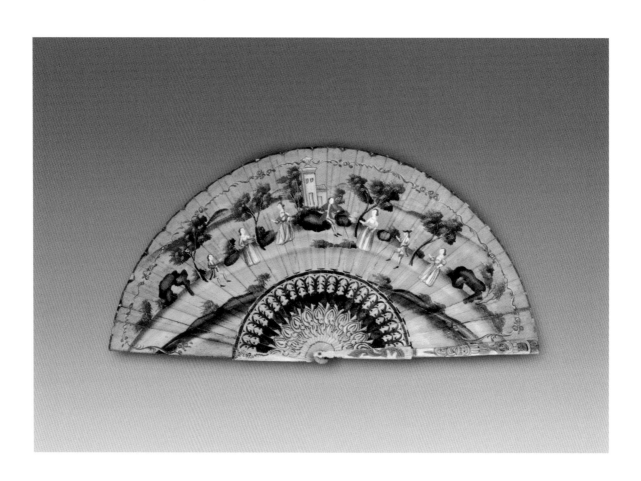

象牙人物扇

清

象牙质

宽 53.8 厘米

Ivory Fan with Western Figures

Qing Dynasty

Ivory

Width 53.8 cm

象牙骨折扇。在扇两面彩绘西欧风情人物画，

工艺精细，是珍贵的工艺美术作品。

沙巴治藏

The fan is an ivory folding fan. Both sides of

the fan are colored with drawings of Western

European style portraits. The handicraft is

exquisite and one of the precious arts and crafts.

Collected by Shabazhi

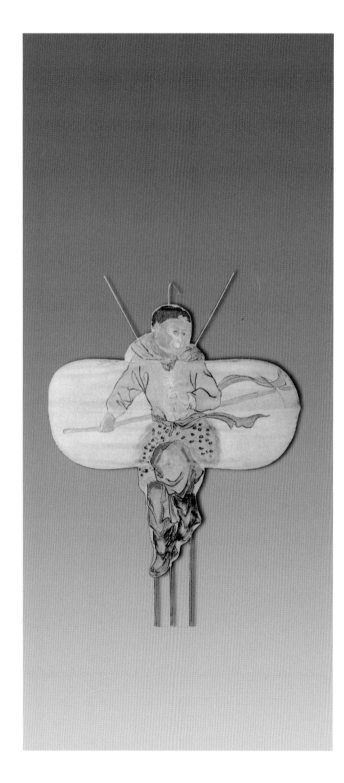

孙悟空风筝

清

木质

宽 70 厘米，高 70 厘米

Kite with Monkey King Image

Qing Dynasty

Wood

Width 70 cm/ Height 70 cm

风筝以《西游记》中孙悟空为原型设计而成，

造型别致，颇具特色。

　　　　　　　潍坊世界风筝博物馆藏

The design of the kite is based on the prototype of the Monkey King in *the Journey to the West*. It is unique in shape with distinctive characteristics.

Preserved in the World Kite Museum in Weifang

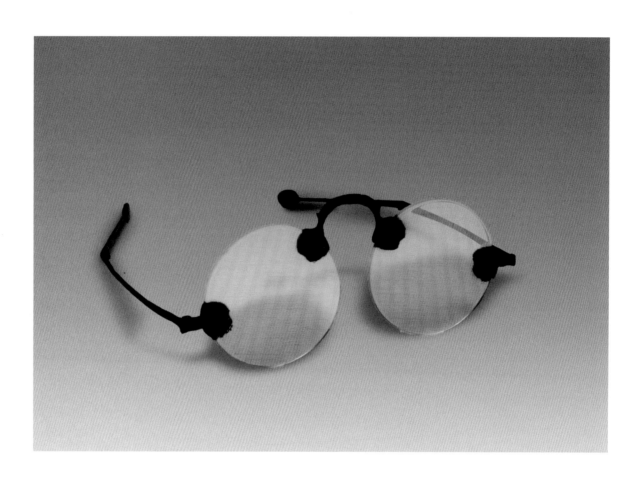

眼镜

清

铜质、玻璃质

镜片直径为 4.5 厘米，架长 13 厘米，宽 11.5 厘米

Glasses

Qing Dynasty

Bronze and Glass

Lens Diameter 4.5 cm/ Frame Length 13 cm/ Width 11.5 cm

铜质镜架，锈蚀严重，柄中间有枢钮，可折叠，玻璃镜片由民间征集。

成都中医药大学中医药传统文化博物馆

The glasses are badly rusted and corroded. The hinge between the two legs is foldable and has glass sheet. It was collected from a private owner.

Preserved in Museum of Traditional Chinese Medicine Culture, Chengdu University of Traditional Chinese Medicine

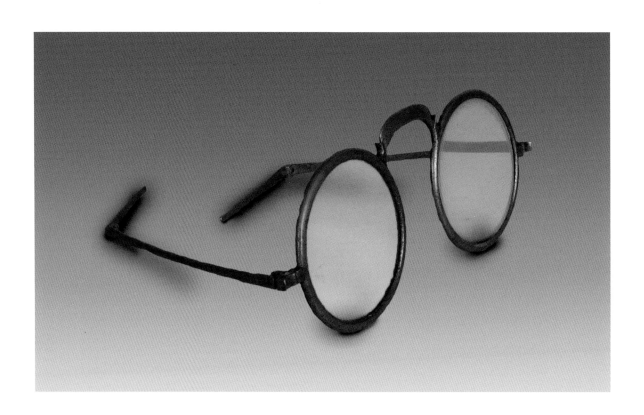

折叠眼镜

清

铜质、玻璃质

镜长 12.9 厘米，镜宽 5 厘米

腿长 13 厘米

Folding Glasses

Qing Dynasty

Bronze and Glass

Frame Length 12.9 cm/ Frame Width 5 cm.

Legs Length 13 cm

该藏是无色老花镜，镜腿为直形折叠式，黄铜镜架，玻璃镜片制成。本物是校正视力用具。1963 年入藏。

中华医学会 / 上海中医药大学医史博物馆藏

The collection is colorless presbyopic glasses. The brass frame legs are straight and foldable. With a bronze frame and glass sheet The glasses were utilized for correcting vision and were collected in 1963.

Preserved in Chinese Medical Association/ Museum of Chinese Medicine, Shanghai University of Traditional Chinese Medicine

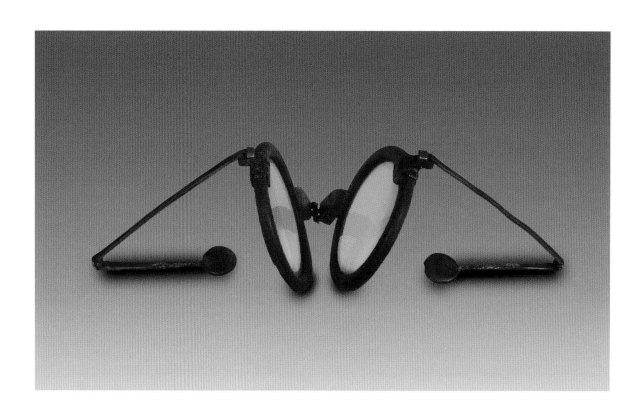

折叠眼镜

清

角质、玻璃质

镜长 14 厘米，镜宽 6.4 厘米

腿长 12.8 厘米

Folding Glasses

Qing Dynasty

Horn and Glass

Frame Length 14 cm/ Frame Width 6.4 cm

Legs Length 12.8 cm

该藏是无色老花镜，镜腿为直形折叠式，金属制成，镜片框为角质，镜片为玻璃质。该藏是校正视力用具。1963 年入藏。

中华医学会 / 上海中医药大学医史博物馆藏

The collection is colorless presbyopic glasses. The metal legs are straight and foldable. The frame is made of horn and has a glass sheet and. The glasses were utilized for correcting vision and were collected in 1963.

Preserved in Chinese Medical Association/ Museum of Chinese Medicine, Shanghai University of Traditional Chinese Medicine

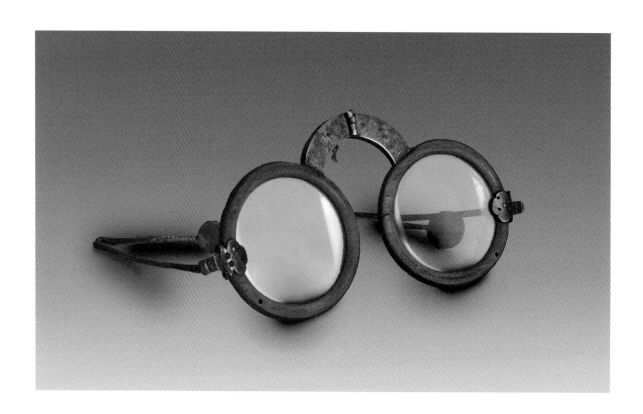

折叠眼镜

清

角质、玻璃质

镜长 14 厘米，镜宽 6.4 厘米

腿长 12.8 厘米

Folding Glasses

Qing Dynasty

Horn and Glass

Frame Length 14 cm/ Frame Width 6.4 cm

Legs Length 12.8 cm

该藏是无色老花镜，镜腿为直形折叠式，金属制成，镜片框为角质，镜片为玻璃质。该藏是校正视力用具。1963 年入藏。

中华医学会 / 上海中医药大学医史博物馆藏

The collection is colorless presbyopic glasses. The metal legs are straight and foldable. The frame is made of horn and the glass sheet is made of glass. The glasses were utilized for correcting vision and were collected in 1963. Preserved in Chinese Medical Association/ Museum of Chinese Medicine, Shanghai University of Traditional Chinese Medicine

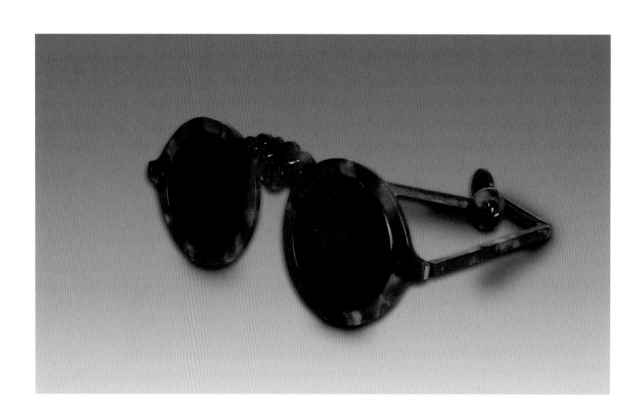

茶晶眼镜

清

塑料质、玻璃质

镜长 13.5 厘米，镜宽 5.2 厘米

腿长 14 厘米

Dark Brown Citrine Sunglasses

Qing Dynasty

Plastic and Glass

Frame Length 13.5 cm/ Frame Width 5.2 cm

Legs Length 14 cm

眼镜形。该藏是茶色太阳镜，镜腿为直形折
叠式，塑料镜架，金属托条，玻璃镜片。本
物为用具，1955 年入藏。

中华医学会 / 上海中医药大学医史博物馆藏

The collection is a pair of dark brown citrine
sunglass. The frame legs are straight and
foldable with a plastic frame, a metal base strip
and glass sheet. They were for daily use and
were collected in 1955.

Preserved in Chinese Medical Association/
Museum of Chinese Medicine, Shanghai
University of Traditional Chinese Medicine

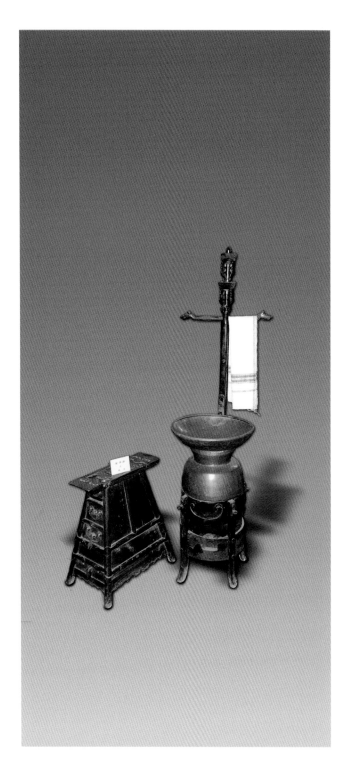

剃头担子

清

铜质、木质

凳高 46 厘米，盆直径 23 厘米，通高 124 厘米

Mobile Combination Tools for Head Shaving

Qing Dynasty

Bronze and Wood

Stool Height 46 cm/ Bronze Basin Diameter 23 cm/

Height 124 cm

铜炉1件，铜脸盆1件，木支架1件，坐椅1件，手巾1件。基本完整。陕西省礼泉县征集。

陕西医史博物馆藏

The combined set consists of a bronze stove, a bronze basin, a wooden support, a stool and a hand towel. They were collected in Li Quan, Shaanxi Province and are almost intact.

Preserved in Shaanxi Museum of Medicine History

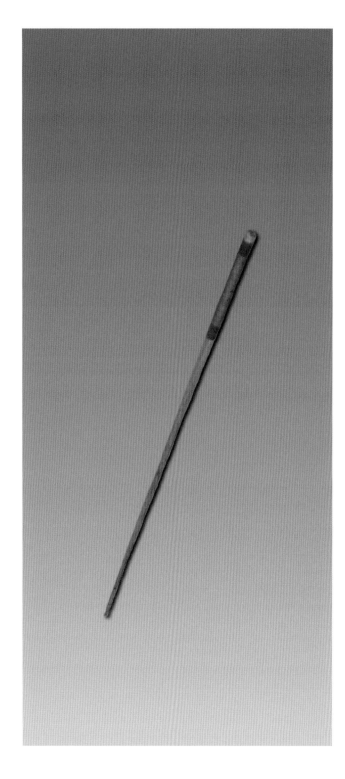

清理耳鼻工具

清

竹质

柄径 0.3 厘米，通长 17 厘米

Ear and Nose Clean-up Tool

Qing Dynasty

Bamboo

Diameter 0.3 cm/ Length 17 cm

长条形。这是该馆通过自购收藏的清末理发用卫生工具之一。这种工具常用作清洁耳鼻内污物。为卫生用具。保存基本完好。

中华医学会 / 上海中医药大学医史博物馆藏

The tool is in the shape of a thin stick. It was one of the sanitary appliances in the late Qing Dynasty. This sanitary tool was utilized for cleaning up the earwax and booger and is still in good condition.

Preserved in Chinese Medical Association/ Museum of Chinese Medicine, Shanghai University of Traditional Chinese Medicine

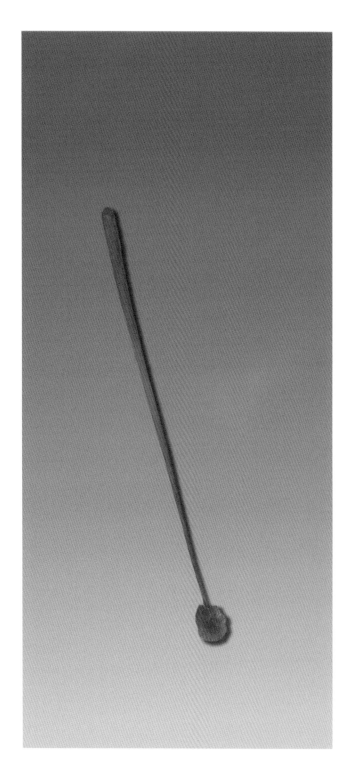

清理耳鼻工具

清

角质

柄径 0.5 厘米，通长 19 厘米

Ear and Nose Clean-up Tool

Qing Dynasty

Horn

Handle Diameter 0.5 cm/ Length 19 cm

长条形。这是该馆通过自购收藏的清末理发
用卫生工具之一。这种工具常用作清洁耳鼻
内污物。为卫生用具。保存基本完好。

中华医学会 / 上海中医药大学医史博物馆藏

The tool is in the shape of a thin stick. It was
one of the sanitary appliances in the late Qing
Dynasty. This sanitary tool was utilized for
cleaning up the earwax and booger and is still
in good condition.

Preserved in Chinese Medical Association/
Museum of Chinese Medicine, Shanghai
University of Traditional Chinese Medicine

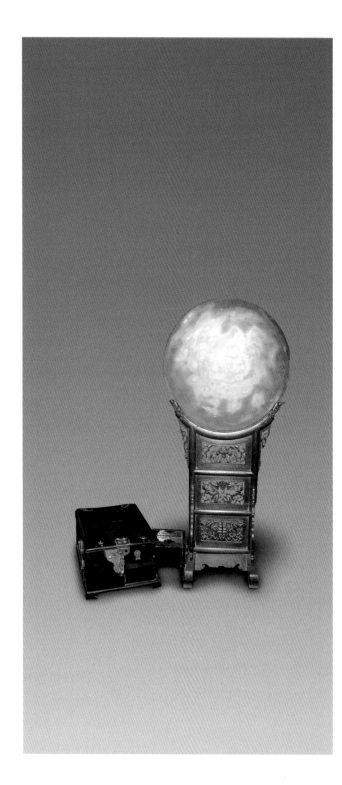

梳妆盒和铜镜

清

铜质、木质

铜镜：直径 37 厘米，高 85 厘米

梳妆盒：长 28 厘米，宽 19 厘米

Dressing Case and Bronze Mirror

Qing Dynasty

Bronze and Wood

Bronze Mirror: Diameter 37 cm/ Height 85 cm

Dressing Case: Length 28 cm/ Width 19 cm

漆木梳妆盒 1 件，内有大小不等的多个小抽屉，圆形铜镜 1 件，楠木铜镜支架 1 件。卫生器具。1997 年入藏，完整无损。陕西省咸阳市征集。

陕西医史博物馆藏

The set contains one lacquer dressing case with various size drawers inside, one round bronze mirror and a nanmu wooden mirror support. The set is a sanitary ware. It was collected in 1997 in Xianyang City, Shaanxi Province. The whole set is intact and in good condition.

Preserved in Shaanxi Museum of Medicine History

象牙镂雕人物塔式瓶

清

象牙质

高 58.5 厘米，口径 11.2~12.5 厘米，底径 9.2~10.2 厘米

象牙瓶为塔式，瓶为传世品，由盖和瓶身分多层组合而成，配置于嵌银丝海梅座上瓶颈两侧对称雕有兽面，瑞兽口衔一只可活动套环。象牙瓶采用镂雕、浅刻、微刻等多种技法，刀工见棱见角，做工精细规矩。通体以人物、花卉、楼台亭榭和园林风光为主，间以缠枝纹、仰莲瓣纹、回纹等辅助纹饰层加以分隔。具有清代晚期广东牙雕的风格和特点。

扬州博物馆藏

Tower-type Ivory Bottle Carved with Figures in Openwork

Qing Dynasty

Ivory

Height 58.5 cm/ Mouth Diameter 11.2 ~12.5 cm/ Bottom Diameter 9.2 ~10.2 cm

The ivory bottle is shaped as a tower. The bottle is a treasure handed down from ancient times. It consists of a lid and a body assembled with multi-layers. The bottle is set on a Haimei-wood base which is inlaid with silver wire. Two beast-face images are symmetrically engraved on both sides of the bottle neck. Each of their mouths has a movable ring. Many different engraving techniques are utilized, including openwork, low relief, and micro-engraving. The knife skills and craftsmanship are exquisite. The entire bottle is engraved mainly with figures, flowers, towers, pavilions, gardens and parks, separated with auxiliary ornamentation layers, such as twine patterns, lotus-petal patterns and meandering patterns. The whole item has the typical styles and characteristics of Guangdong ivory engraving in the late Qing Dynasty.

Preserved in Yangzhou Museum

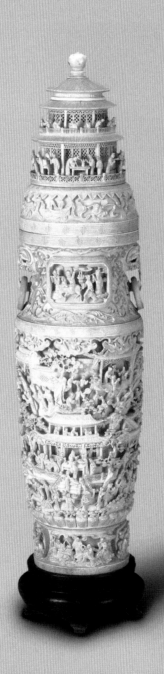

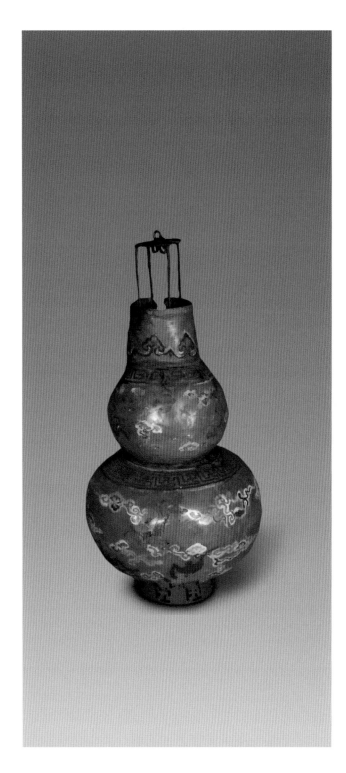

葫芦灯笼

清

塑料质、铁质

宽 21 厘米，通高 43 厘米

Gourd-shaped Lantern

Qing Dynasty

Plastic and Iron Wire

Width 21 cm/ Height 43 cm

葫芦形。灯笼罩用塑料制成，以长铁丝连接底座和顶，葫芦形灯罩表面绘蝙蝠、祥云图案。为灯具。1958 年入藏。

中华医学会 / 上海中医药大学医史博物馆藏

The lantern cover is made of plastic. A long iron wire links the lantern from its pedestal to top. The gourd-shaped cover is painted with designs and patterns of bats and auspicious clouds. The gourd-shaped lantern was utilized as a lamp. It was collected in 1958.

Preserved in Chinese Medical Association/ Museum of Chinese Medicine, Shanghai University of Traditional Chinese Medicine

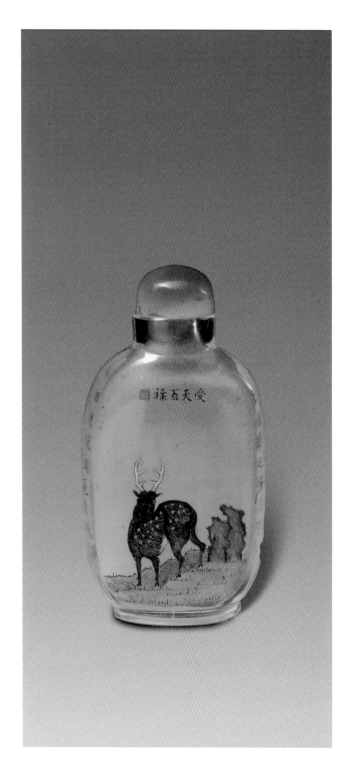

马少宣绘受天百禄图料烟壶

清

玻璃质

口径 1.5 厘米，宽 3.5 厘米，厚 1.2 厘米，
高 6.3 厘米

Glass Snuff Bottle

Qing Dynasty

Glass

Mouth Diameter 1.5 cm/ Width 3.5 cm/

Thickness 1.2 cm/ Height 6.3 cm

烟壶呈扁圆形。正面绘《受天百禄图》，一鹿伫立山坡，翘首张望。背面楷书节录王羲之《兰亭序》，落款"马少宣"。

山东省潍坊市文物商店藏

The bottle is in an oblate form. The obverse side is carved with Shou Tian Bai Lu Tu. A deer is standing on the hillside raising their heads and looking around. The reverse side is the excerpts of "Lanting Xu" written by Wang Xizhi in regular script. The inscription "Ma Shaoxuan" is carved on the bottle.

Preserved in the Antique Store of Weifang, Shandong Province

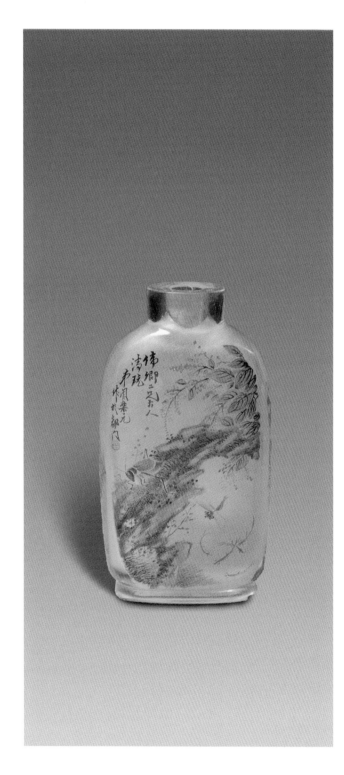

周乐元绘柳荫垂钓料烟壶

清

玻璃质

口径 1.5 厘米，宽 3.5 厘米，厚 1.2 厘米，

高 6.3 厘米

Glass Snuff Bottle with Design of Fishing under Willow Tree

Qing Dynasty

Glass

Mouth Diameter 1.5cm/ Width 3.5 cm/

Thickness 1.2 cm/ Height 6.3 cm

料烟壶呈扁圆形。正面绘柳荫垂钓图，远处山影隐约可见，近处柳荫下一老翁泊舟垂钓。背面画有怪石花草，蝈蝈静立其上，蜻蜓振翅翻飞，一静一动，相映成趣。画面左方有周乐元题款。

山东省潍坊市文物商店藏

The bottle has an oblate body. The obverse side is a painting of a man fishing under the willow shadows. The distant hill shade is indistinct; and an old man in a small boat is fishing under a willow tree. The reverse side is painted with strange rocks, flowers, and grass on which a grasshopper stands still and a dragonfly is fluttering up and down. The sharp contrast between the motionless grasshopper and the moving dragonfly make the picture vivid, delightful and beautiful. The left side of the picture is the inscription Zhou Leyuan.

Preserved in the Antique Store of Weifang City Shandong Province

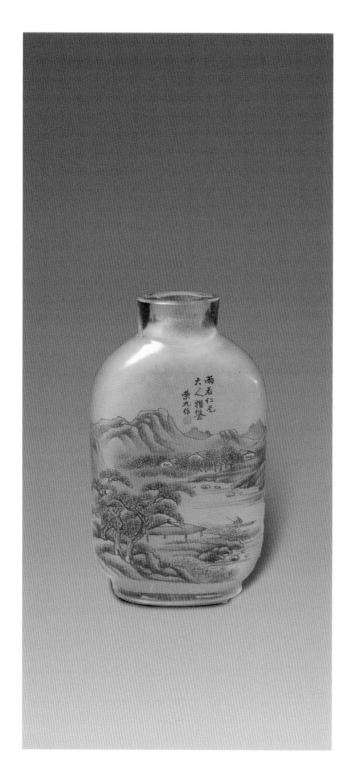

毕荣九绘山水料烟壶

清

玻璃质

口径 1.7 厘米，宽 3.8 厘米，厚 1.8 厘米，

高 6 厘米

Glass Snuff Bottle Drawn with Landscape by Bi Rongjiu

Qing Dynasty

Glass

Mouth Diameter 1.7 cm/ Width 3.8 cm/

Thickness 1.8 cm/ Height 6 cm

料烟壶呈扁圆形。正背两面为一幅完整的山水画，山岭逶迤，山脚下万树丛中隐现几栋农舍。溪水汩汩，在山下聚成一泓清潭，潭中渔者泛舟。傍水一条小径，弯弯曲曲隐入山中。整幅画面充满恬静的田园情趣。

山东省潍坊市文物商店藏

The bottle has an oblate body. Paintings on both sides form a complete landscape. The winding mountains are in the distance and several farm houses can be seen indistinctly in the forests at the foot of the mountain. The rippling streams flow together at the foot of the mountain and form a deep pool, where a fisherman is rowing his boat. Along the waterside, a pathway zigzags into the mountains. The entire view is full of tranquil and peaceful pastoralism.

Preserved in the Antique Store of Weifang, Shandong Province

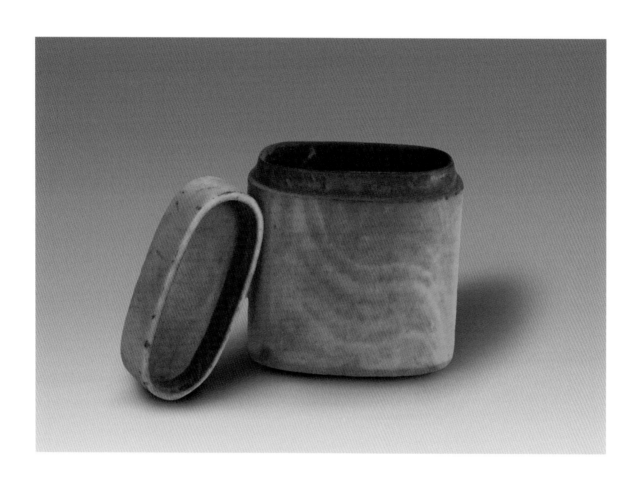

烟盒

清

象牙质

宽 4.4 厘米，厚 2.05 厘米，通高 5.04 厘米

Tobacco Box

Qing Dynasty

Ivory

Width 4.4 cm/ Thickness 2.05 cm/ Height 5.04 cm

扁瓶状，烟具。该藏通体磨光，牙质泛黄，

盒内呈黑色。用于存烟。1955 年入藏，保存

完好。

中华医学会 / 上海中医药大学医史博物馆藏

The box is shaped as a flat bottle and is a
smoking set. The box is polished entirely. The
ivory is yellowing and the interior color of the
box is black. It was utilized for storing tobacco.
It was collected in 1955 and is still in good
condition.

Preserved in Chinese Medical Association/
Museum of Chinese Medicine, Shanghai
University of Traditional Chinese Medicine

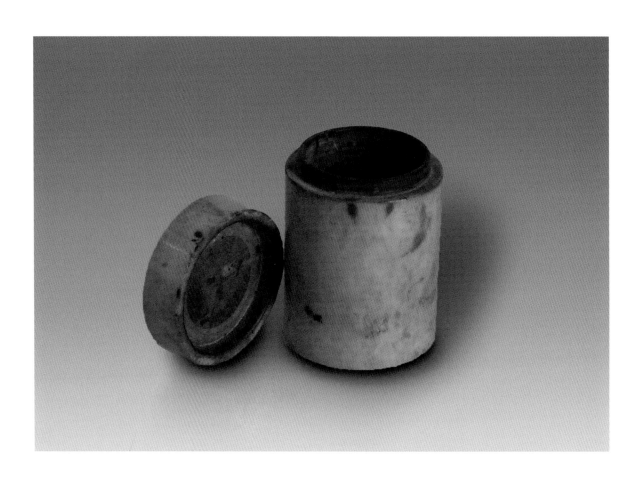

烟盒

清

象牙质

直径 3.05 厘米，通高 4.45 厘米

Tobacco Box

Qing Dynasty

Ivory

Diameter 3.05 cm/ Height 4.45 cm

圆筒状。该藏通体磨光，牙质泛黄，盒内呈
黑色。烟具。1955 年入藏，保存完好。

中华医学会／上海中医药大学医史博物馆藏

The box is shaped as a cylindrical bottle. The
box is polished entirely. The ivory is yellowing
and the interior color of the box is black. It was
utilized for storing tobacco. It was collected in
1955 and is still in good condition.

Preserved in Chinese Medical Association/
Museum of Chinese Medicine, Shanghai
University of Traditional Chinese Medicine

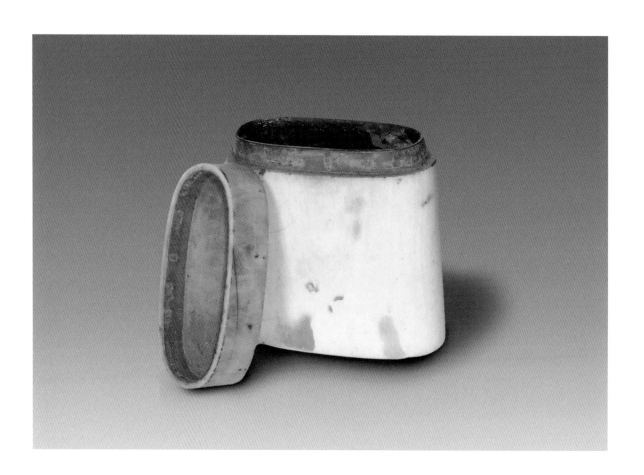

烟盒

清

象牙质

宽 4.4 厘米，厚 2.05 厘米，通高 5.04 厘米

Tobacco Box

Qing Dynasty

Ivory

Width 4.4 cm/ Thickness 2.05 cm/ Height 5.04 cm

扁瓶状。该藏用于存烟，通体磨光，牙质泛黄，

盒内呈黑色。烟具。1955 年入藏，保存完好。

中华医学会 / 上海中医药大学医史博物馆藏

The box is shaped as a flat bottle and is a
smoking set. The box is polished entirely. The
ivory is yellowing and the interior color of the
box is black. It was utilized for storing tobacco.
It was collected in 1955 and is still in good
condition.

Preserved in Chinese Medical Association/
Museum of Chinese Medicine, Shanghai
University of Traditional Chinese Medicine

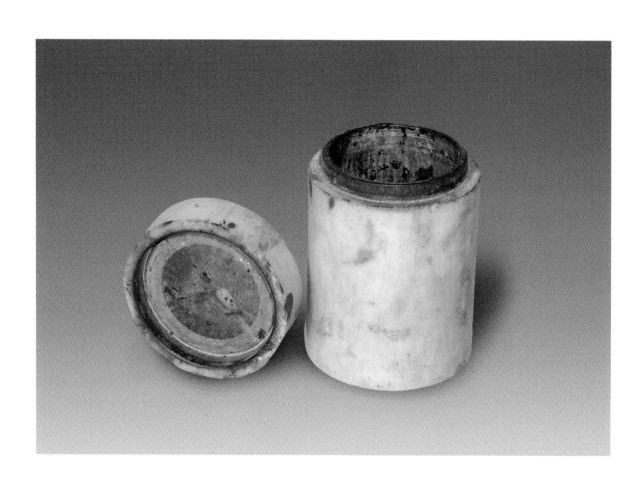

烟盒

清

象牙质

直径 3.05 厘米，通高 4.45 厘米

Tobacco Box

Qing Dynasty

Ivory

Diameter 3.05 cm/ Height 4.45 cm

圆筒状。该藏瓶身通体磨光，牙质泛黄，盒内呈黑色。烟具。1955 年入藏，保存完好。

中华医学会 / 上海中医药大学医史博物馆藏

The box is shaped as a cylindrical bottle. The box is polished entirely. The ivory is yellowing and the interior color of the box is black. It was utilized for storing tobacco. It was collected in 1955 and is still in good condition.

Preserved in Chinese Medical Association/ Museum of Chinese Medicine, Shanghai University of Traditional Chinese Medicine

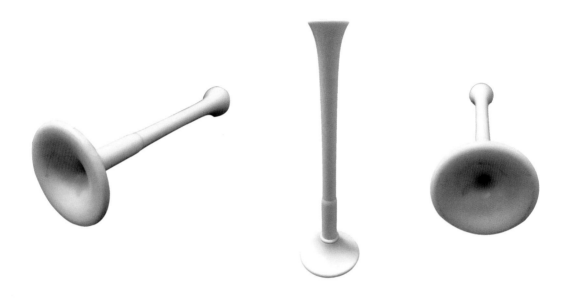

象牙听诊器

清

骨质

长 18 厘米，大口直径 5 厘米，小口直径 2~3 厘米

Ivory Echoscope

Qing dynasty

Bone

Length 18 cm/ Large Mouth Diameter 5 cm/ Small Mouth Diameter 2~3 cm

素面，诊疗器具，小口置于医生耳部，大口
放于听诊部位。

新昌县天姥中医博物馆藏

The surface of the echoscope has no decorations.
It was utilized to diagnose diseases by putting
the smaller mouth in doctor's ears and the bigger
mouth on the diagnostic part of patients' body.
Preserved in Tianmu Traditional Chinese Medicine
Museum of Xinchang County

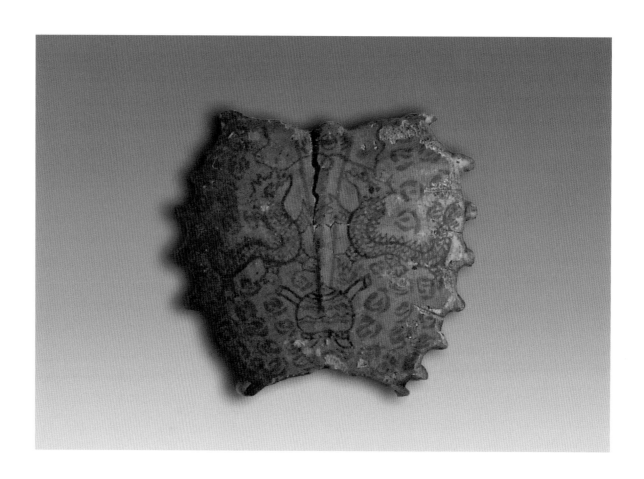

辟邪龟甲

清

龟甲质

长 11.5 厘米，宽 12.5 厘米

Tortoise Shell for Counteracting Evil Force

Qing Dynasty

Tortoise shell

Length 11.5 cm/ Width 12.5 cm

龟背形。为神符。该神符用龟甲制成，一面绘有双龙和香熏图案；内面粘有布片，上写有文字和图案，内容辨别不清。1955年入藏，保存基本完好，中部有裂缝。

中华医学会／上海中医药大学医史博物馆藏

The collection, a kind of hierogram, is shaped as a turtleback. The hierogram is made of tortoise shell. Paintings of two dragons and fragrant designs are carved on one side of the shell. Pieces of cloth are stuck to the other side but the characters and designs on the cloth are indecipherable. It was collected in 1955 and is almost in good conditions, only with a crack at the central part.

Preserved in Chinese Medical Association/ Museum of Chinese Medicine, Shanghai University of Traditional Chinese Medicine

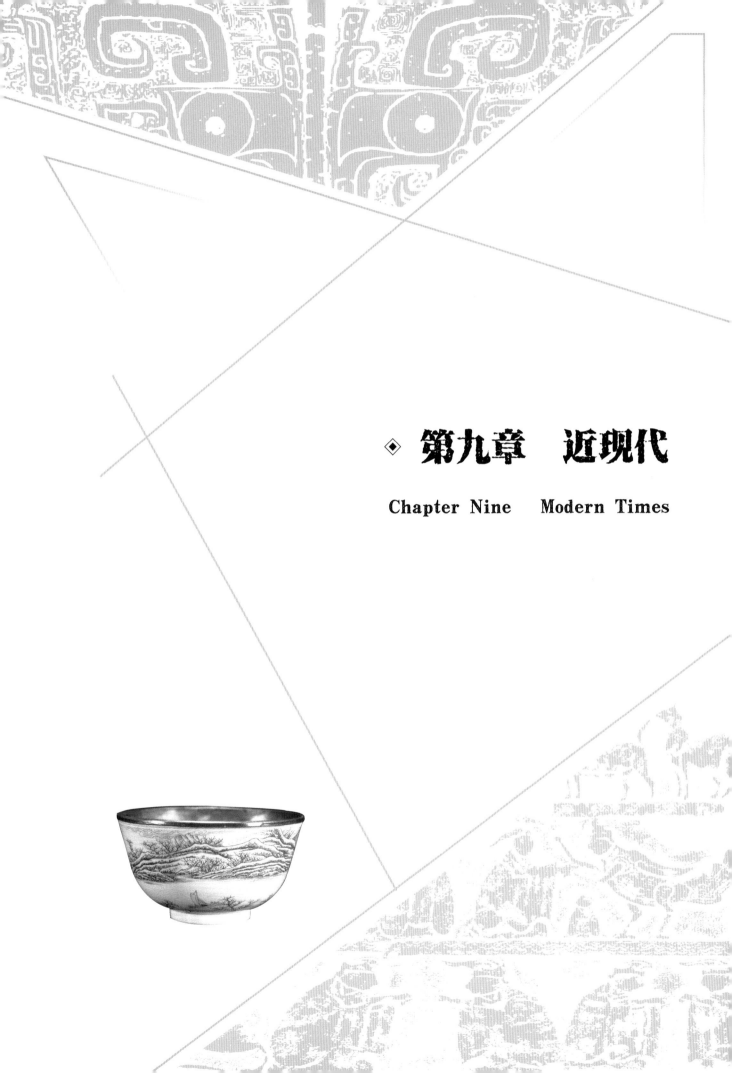

◈ 第九章　近现代

Chapter Nine　Modern Times

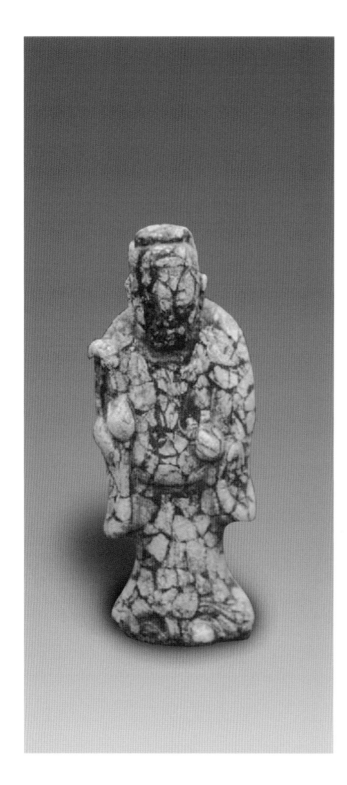

雄精雕刻吕祖像

近代

矿物质

长 5.7 厘米，宽 3 厘米，通高 14.4 厘米，
重 28 克

Realgar Statue of Lu Dongbin

Modern Times

Mineral

Length 5.7 cm/ Width 3 cm/ Height 14.4 cm/

Weight 28 g

雄精即雄黄，是一种中药。此是用中药材雕刻的
人物塑像。

广东中医药博物馆藏

Realgar is a kind of Traditional Chinese Medicine.
The figure statue is carved with this Chinese herbal
medicine.

Preserved in Guangzhou Chinese Medicine Museum

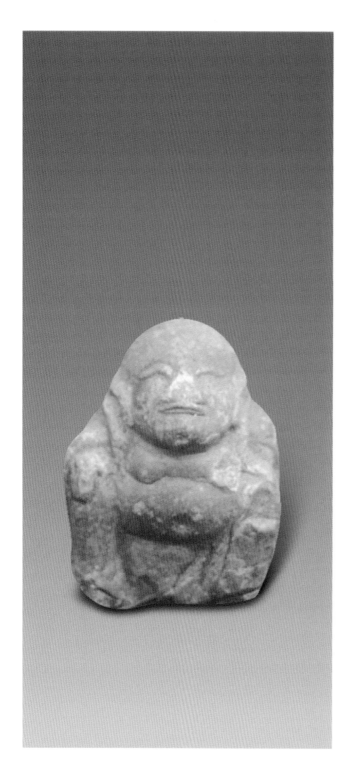

雄精雕刻

近代

矿物质

长 3.6 厘米，宽 2.75 厘米，通高 4.5 厘米，
重 76 克

Realgar Carving

Modern Times

Mineral

Length 3.6 cm/ Width 2.75 cm/ Height 4.5 cm/
Weight 76 g

雄精即雄黄，是一种中药，此为雄黄雕刻的艺术品。用于装饰，并有避邪的作用。

广东中医药博物馆藏

The Realgar is a kind of Traditional Chinese Medicine. The collection is an artwork of realgar carving. It was utilized for decoration and also for avoiding evil spirits.

Preserved in Guangzhou Chinese Medicine Museum

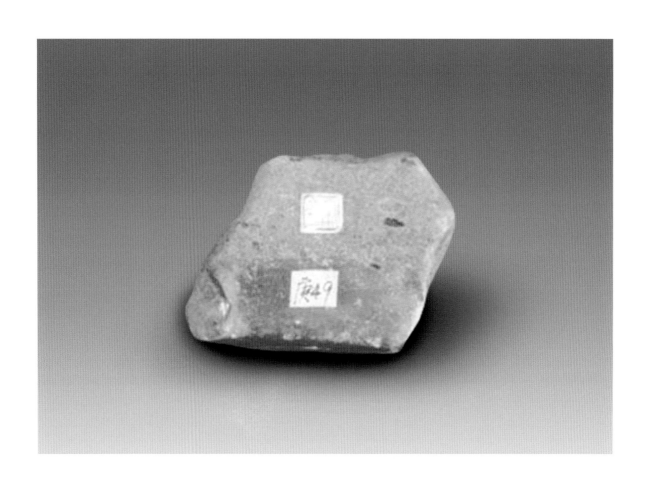

雄精雕刻

近代

矿物质

长 5.2 厘米，宽 1.35 厘米，通高 3.2 厘米，重 50 克

Realgar Carving

Modern Times

Mineral

Length 5.2 cm/ Width 1.35 cm/ Height 3.2 cm/ Weight 50 g

雄精即雄黄，是一种中药，此为雄黄雕刻的艺术
品，用于装饰，并有避邪的作用。

广东中医药博物馆藏

Realgar is a kind of traditional Chinese medicine.
The collection is an artwork of realgar carving. It
was utilized for decoration and for avoiding evil
spirits.

Preserved in Guangzhou Chinese Medicine Museum

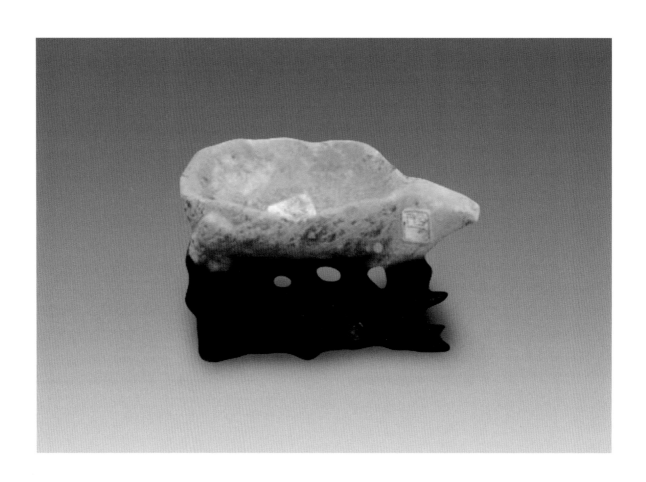

雄精雕刻

近代

矿物质

长 7.4 厘米，宽 4.6 厘米，通高 2.1 厘米，重 82 克

Realgar Carving

Modern Times

Mineral

Length 7.4 cm/ Width 4.6 cm/ Height 2.1 cm/ Weight 82 g

雄精即雄黄，是一种中药，此为雄黄雕刻的艺术

品，用于装饰，并有避邪的作用。

广东中医药博物馆藏

Realgar is a kind of traditional Chinese medicine.
The collection is an artwork of realgar carving. It
was utilized for decoration and for avoiding evil
spirits.

Preserved in Guangzhou Chinese Medicine Museum

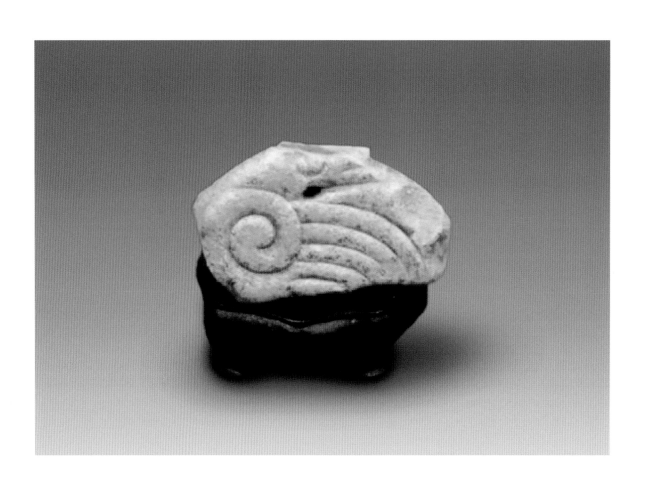

雄精雕刻

近代

矿物质

长 3.5 厘米，宽 1.35 厘米，通高 1.9 厘米，重 15 克

Realgar Carving

Modern Times

Mineral

Length 3.5 cm/ Width 1.35 cm/ Height 1.9 cm/ Weight 15 g

雄黄制，一种中药材雕刻的艺术品。用于装饰，
并有避邪的作用。

广东中医药博物馆藏

Realgar is a kind of traditional Chinese medicine.
The collection is an artwork of realgar carving. It
was utilized for decoration and for avoiding evil
spirits.

Preserved in Guangzhou Chinese Medicine Museum

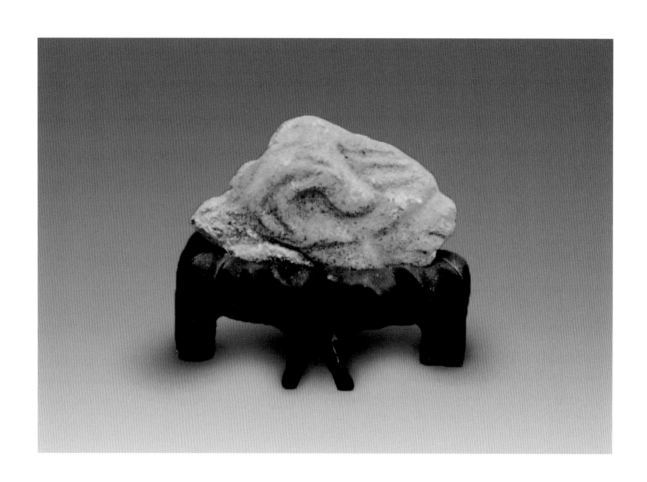

雄精雕刻

近代

矿物质

长 4.85 厘米，宽 2 厘米，通高 3.1 厘米，重 42 克

Realgar Carving

Modern Times

Mineral

Length 4.85 cm/ Width 2 cm/ Height 3.1 cm/ Weight 42 g

雄精即雄黄，是一种中药，此为雄黄雕刻的艺术品。用于装饰，并有避邪的作用。

广东中医药博物馆藏

Realgar is a kind of traditional Chinese medicine. The collection is an artwork of realgar carving. It was utilized for decoration and for avoiding evil spirits.

Preserved in Guangzhou Chinese Medicine Museum

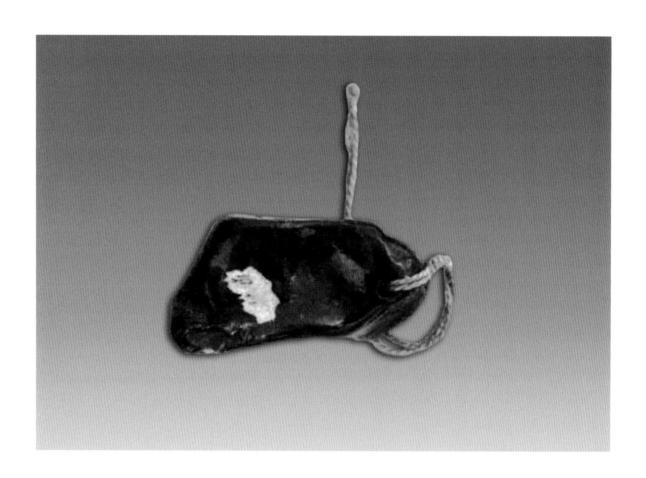

天然形琥珀

近代

化石

长 2.3 厘米，宽 1.7 厘米，通高 5.2 厘米，重 11 克

Amber in Natural Shape

Modern Times

Fossil

Length 2.3 cm/ Width 1.7 cm/ Height 5.2 cm/ Weight 11 g

琥珀是松柏树脂的化石，可入药，也可制成饰物。
此为琥珀制的一种饰物。

广东中医药博物馆藏

Amber is the fossil of resin from cypress and pine
trees. It could be utilized for medicine and be made
into ornaments. This is an amber-made ornament.
Preserved in Guangzhou Chinese Medicine Museum

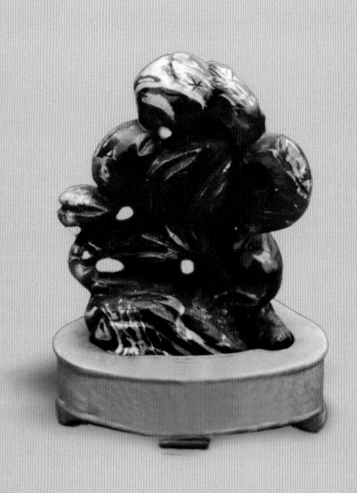

琥珀雕寿桃摆件

近代

化石

长 6.5 厘米， 宽 2.9 厘米， 通高 9.25 厘米（带底座），
重 94 克

琥珀是松柏树脂的化石，可入药，亦可制成饰物。此
为琥珀制的寿桃摆件，用于装饰。

广东中医药博物馆藏

Amber Carved in the Shape of Peach Tree

Modern Times

Fossil

Length 6.5 cm/ Width 2.9 cm/ Height 9.25 cm (with the base)/
Weight 94 g

Amber is the fossil of resin from cypress and pine
trees. It could be utilized as medicine and be made into
ornaments. This is an amber-made ornament of peach-
shaped birthday cake.

Preserved in Guangzhou Chinese Medicine Museum

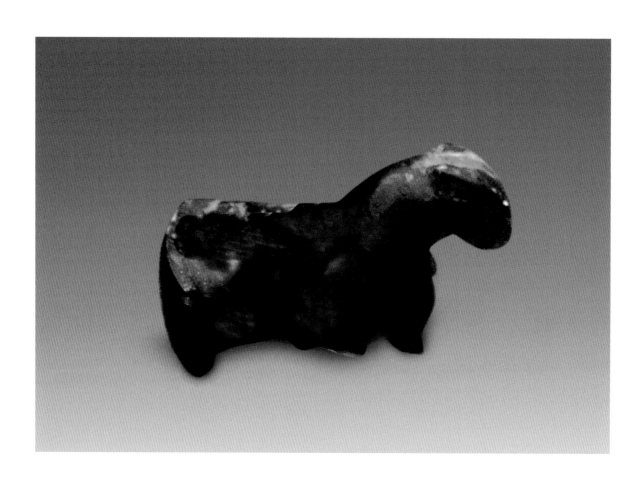

琥珀马形

近代

化石

长 6.75 厘米，高 9 厘米，重 88 克

Horse-shaped Amber Ornament

Modern Times

Fossil

Length 6.75 cm/ Height 9 cm/ Weight 88 g

琥珀是松柏树脂的化石，可入药，也可制成饰物。
此为琥珀制的一种摆件，马形，用于装饰。

广东中医药博物馆藏

Amber is the fossil of resin from cypress and pine trees. It could be utilized as medicine and be made into ornaments. This is an amber-made and horse-shaped ornament.

Preserved in Guangzhou Chinese Medicine Museum

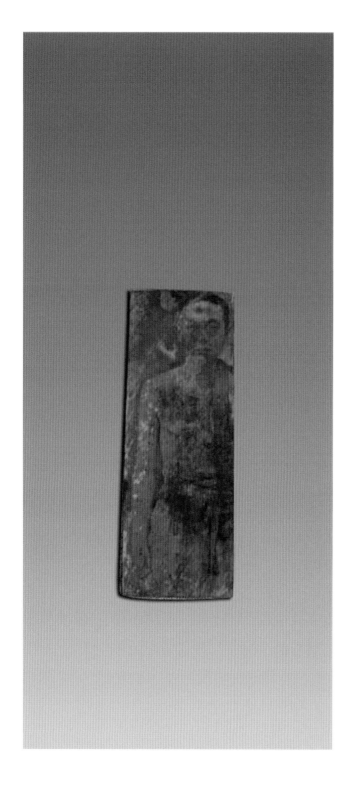

印版

近代

木质、铜质

长 17.5 厘米，宽 6.5 厘米，重 200 克

Printing Plate

Modern Times

Wood and Copper

Length 17.5 cm/ Width 6.5 cm/ Weight 200 g

长方形"手太阴肺径穴图",木质板上粘贴有
一铜版,医药印版。完整无损。陕西省西安市
藻露堂中药店征集。

陕西医史博物馆藏

This rectangle plate is carved with a chart of
"Points of the Lung Meridian of Hand-Taiyin".
A copper plate is stuck to a wooden plate. It was
utilized as a medical printing plate and is still in
good condition. It was collected from Xi'an Zao
Lu Tang Traditional Chinese Medicine Store,
Shaanxi Province.

Preserved in Shaanxi Museum of Medicine History

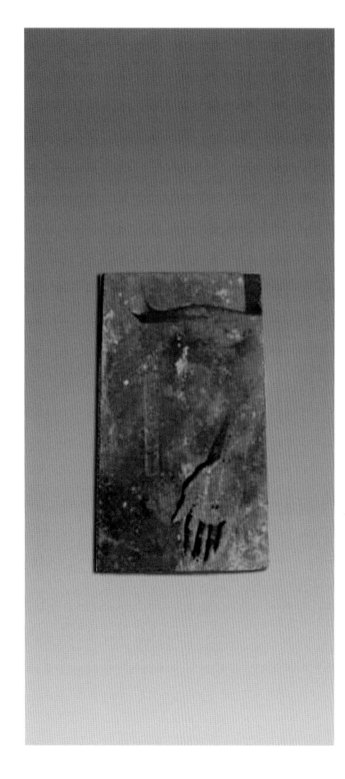

印版

近代

木质、铜质

长 13.2 厘米，宽 7.2 厘米，重 260 克

Printing Plate

Modern Times

Wood and Copper

Length 13.2 cm/ Width 7.2 cm/ Weight 260 g

长方形"手厥阴心包经穴图"，木质板上粘贴有一铜版，医药印版。完整无损。陕西省西安市藻露堂中药店征集。

陕西医史博物馆藏

This rectangle plate is carved with a chart of "Points of the Pericardium Meridian of Hand-Jueyin". A copper plate is stuck to a wooden plate. It was utilized as a medical printing plate and is still in good condition. It was collected from Xi'an Zao Lu Tang Traditional Chinese Medicine Store, Shaanxi Province.

Preserved in Shaanxi Museum of Medicine History

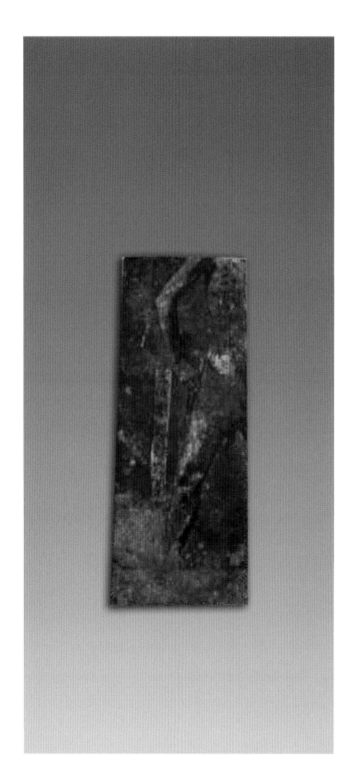

印版

近代

木质、铜质

长 16.5 厘米，宽 6.2 厘米，重 200 克

Printing Plate

Modern Times

Wood and Copper

Length 16.5 cm/ Width 6.2 cm/ Weight 200 g

长方形"足太阴脾经穴图"，木质板上粘贴有
一铜版，医药印版。陕西省西安市藻露堂中药
店征集。完整无损。

陕西医史博物馆藏

The rectangular plate is carved with a chart of
"Points of the Spleen Meridian of Foot-Taiyin".
A copper plate is stuck to a wooden plate. It was
utilized as a medical printing plate and is still in
good condition. It was collected from Xi'an Zao
Lu Tang Traditional Chinese Medicine Store,
Shaanxi Province.

Preserved in Shaanxi Museum of Medicine History

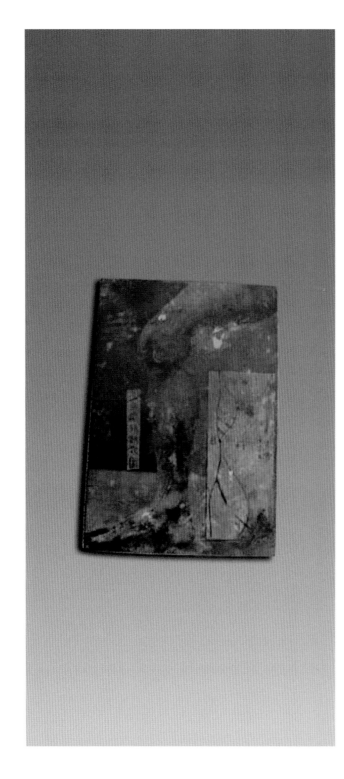

印版

近代

木质、铜质

长 15 厘米，宽 10.5 厘米，重 280 克

Printing Plate

Modern Times

Wood and Copper

Length 15 cm/ Width 10.5 cm/ Weight 280 g

长方形"足厥阴肝经穴图",木质板上粘贴有一铜版,医药印版。陕西省西安市藻露堂中药店征集。完整无损。

陕西医史博物馆藏

The rectangular plate is carved with a chart of "Points of the Liver Meridian of Foot-Jueyin". A copper plate is stuck to a wooden plate. It was utilized as a medical printing plate and is still in good condition. It was collected from Xi'an Zao Lu Tang Traditional Chinese Medicine Store, Shaanxi Province.

Preserved in Shaanxi Museum of Medicine History

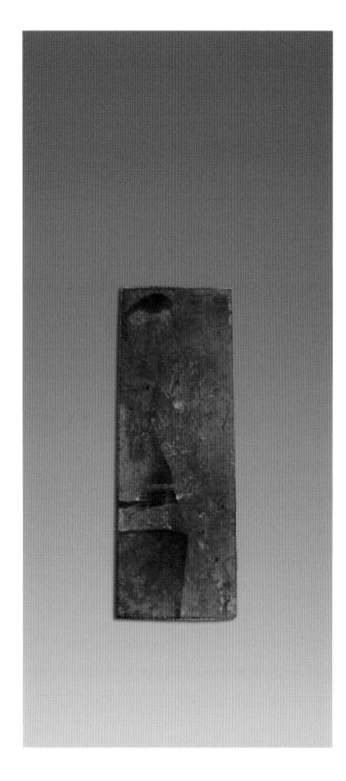

印版

近代

木质、铜质

长 18.5 厘米，宽 6.5 厘米，重 220 克

Printing Plate

Modern Times

Wood and Copper

Length 18.5 cm/ Width 6.5 cm/ Weight 220 g

长方形"手太阳小肠经穴图"，木质板上粘贴有一铜版，医药印版。陕西省西安市藻露堂中药店征集。完整无损。

陕西医史博物馆藏

The rectangular plate is carved with a chart of "Points of the Small Intestines Meridian of Hand-Taiyang". A copper plate is stuck to a wooden plate. It was utilized as a medical printing plate and is still in good condition. It was collected from Xi'an Zao Lu Tang Traditional Chinese Medicine Store, Shaanxi Province.

Preserved in Shaanxi Museum of Medicine History

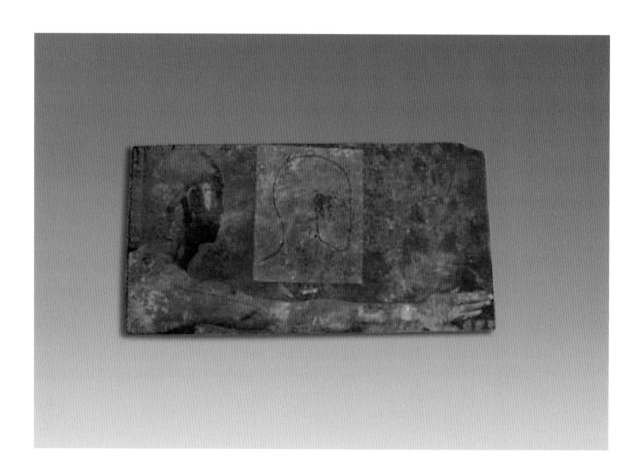

印版

近代

木质、铜质

长 17 厘米，宽 8.5 厘米，重 260 克

Printing Plate

Modern Times

Wood and Copper

Length 17 cm/ Width 8.5 cm/ Weight 260 g

长方形"手少阳三焦经穴图",木质板上粘贴有一铜版,医药印版。陕西省西安市藻露堂中药店征集。完整无损。

陕西医史博物馆藏

The rectangular plate is carved with a chart of "Points of the Triple Energizer Meridian of Hand-shaoyang". A copper plate is stuck to a wooden plate. It was utilized as a medical printing plate and is still in good condition. It was collected from Xi'an Zao Lu Tang Traditional Chinese Medicine Store, Shaanxi Province.

Preserved in Shaanxi Museum of Medicine History

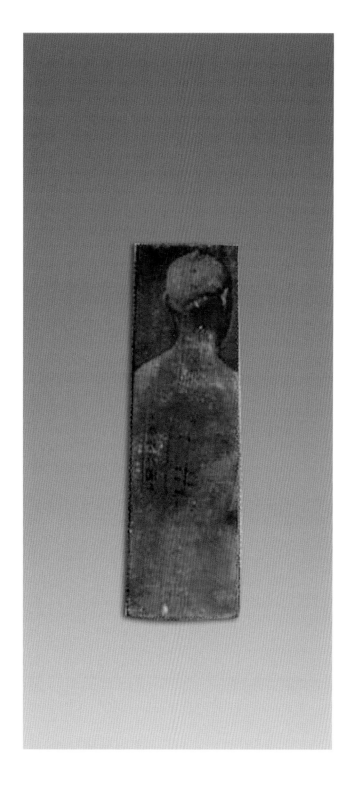

印版

近代

木质、铜质

长 16.2 厘米，宽 4.5 厘米，重 160 克

Printing Plate

Modern Times

Wood and Copper

Length 16.2 cm/ Width 4.5 cm/ Weight 160 g

长方形"足太阳膀胱经穴图"，木质板上粘贴
有一铜版，医药印版。陕西省西安市藻露堂中
药店征集。完整无损。

陕西医史博物馆藏

The rectangular plate is carved with a chart of
"Points of Bladder Meridian of Foot-taiyang".
A copper plate is stuck to a wooden plate. It was
utilized as a medical printing plate and is still in
good condition. It was collected from Xi'an Zao
Lu Tang Traditional Chinese Medicine Store,
Shaanxi Province.

Preserved in Shaanxi Museum of Medicine History

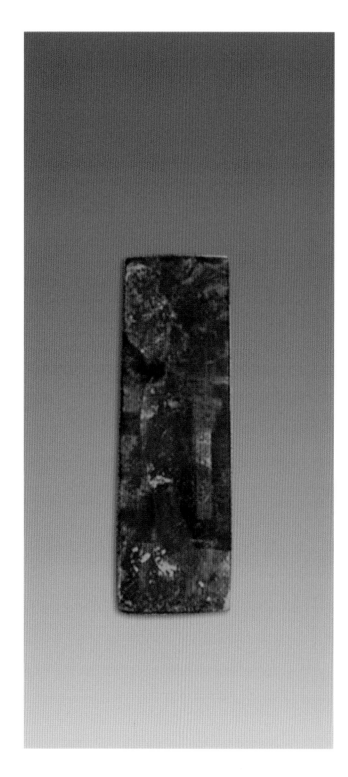

印版

近代

木质、铜质

长 17 厘米，宽 4.4 厘米，重 160 克

Printing Plate

Modern Times

Wood and Copper

Length 17 cm/ Width 4.4 cm/ Weight 160 g

长方形"足阳明胃经穴图",木质板上粘贴有一铜版,医药印版。陕西省西安市藻露堂中药店征集。完整无损。

陕西医史博物馆藏

The rectangular plate is carved with a chart of "Points of Stomach Meridian of Foot-Yangming". A copper plate is stuck to a wooden plate. It was utilized as a medical printing plate and is still in good condition. It was collected from Xi'an Zao Lu Tang Traditional Chinese Medicine Store, Shaanxi Province.

Preserved in Shaanxi Museum of Medicine History

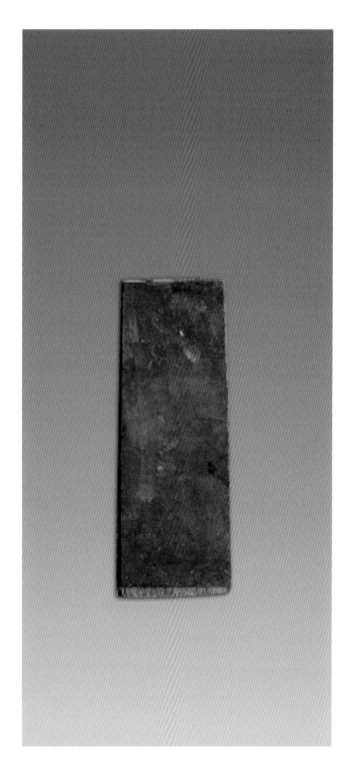

印版

近代

木质、铜质

长 17.5 厘米，宽 6 厘米，重 60 克

Printing Plate

Modern Times

Wood and Copper

Length 17.5 cm/ Width 6 cm/ Weight 60 g

长方形"足少阳胆经穴图",木质板上粘贴有一铜版,医药印版。陕西省西安市藻露堂中药店征集。完整无损。

陕西医史博物馆藏

The rectangular plate is carved with a chart of "Points of the Gallbladder Meridian of Foot-shaoyang". A copper plate is stuck to a wooden plate. It was utilized as a medical printing plate and is still in good condition. It was collected from Xi'an Zao Lu Tang Traditional Chinese Medicine Store, Shaanxi Province.

Preserved in Shaanxi Museum of Medicine History

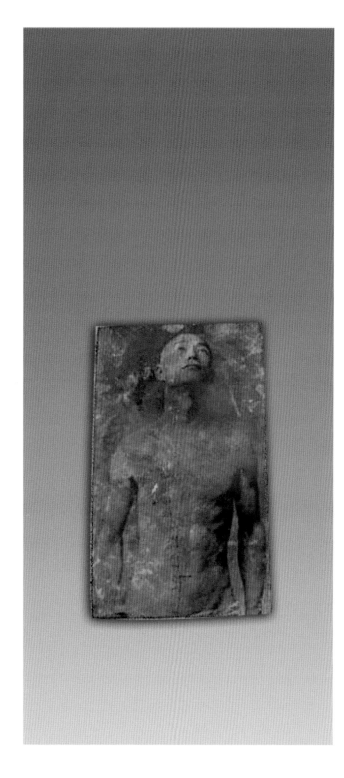

印版

近代

木质、铜质

长 16.5 厘米，宽 10 厘米，重 300 克

Printing Plate

Modern Times

Wood and Copper

Length 16.5 cm/ Width 10 cm/ Weight 300 g

长方形"足少阴肾经穴图",木质板上粘贴有一铜版,医药印版。陕西省西安市藻露堂中药店征集。完整无损。

陕西医史博物馆藏

The rectangular plate is carved with a chart of "Points of the Kidney Meridian of Foot-shaoyin". A copper plate is stuck to a wooden plate. It was utilized as a medical printing plate and is still in good condition. It was collected from Xi'an Zao Lu Tang Traditional Chinese Medicine Store, Shaanxi Province.

Preserved in Shaanxi Museum of Medicine History

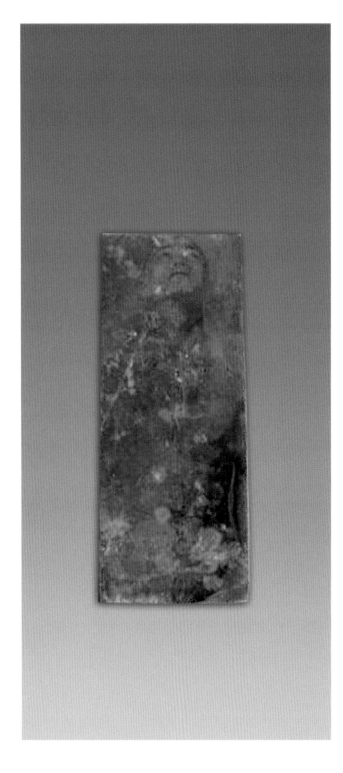

印版

近代

木质、铜质

长 16 厘米，宽 6.3 厘米，重 190 克

Printing Plate

Modern Times

Wood and Copper

Length 16 cm/ Width 6.3 cm/ Weight 190 g

长方形"任脉经穴图",木质板上粘贴有一铜版,

医药印版。陕西省西安市藻露堂中药店征集。

完整无损。

陕西医史博物馆藏

The rectangular plate is carved with a chart of
"Points of the Conception Vessel". A copper
plate is stuck to a wooden plate. It was utilized
as a medical printing plate and is still in good
condition. It was collected from Xi'an Zao Lu
Tang Traditional Chinese Medicine Store, Shaanxi
Province.

Preserved in Shaanxi Museum of Medicine History

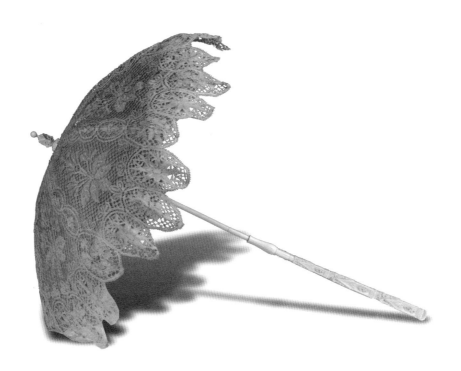

象牙阳伞

近代

象牙质

长 71 厘米

Ivory Parasol

Modern Times

Ivory

Length 71 cm

整把伞都是用象牙雕刻而成，其工艺精美无
比，真可谓广东牙刻一代工艺绝品。

沙巴治藏

The whole parasol is an ivory carving, which
is of exquisite and delicate craftsmanship. It
may be a masterpiece among ivory carvings in
Guangdong.

Collected by Shabazhi

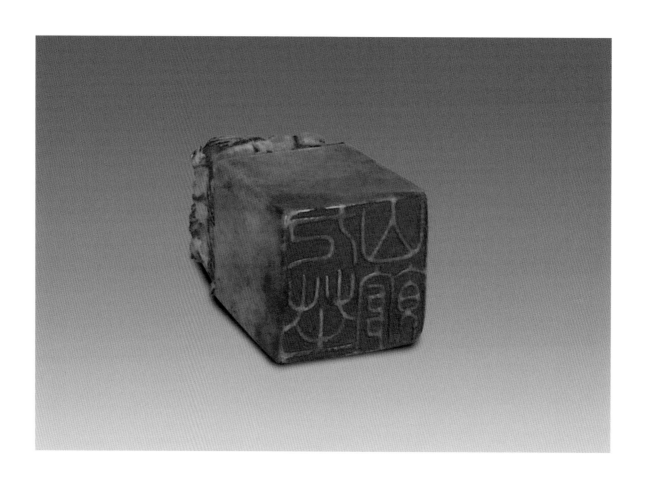

九芝山馆章

近现代

象牙质

边长 2 厘米，高 4.6 厘米

Seal of Jiuzhishanguan

Modern Times

Ivory

Side length 2 cm/ Height 4.6 cm

方形，为私章。该章刻制精细，篆体朱文，形体流畅，印钮为双狮戏球，形态生动。九芝山馆为夏应堂的雅号。1962 年入藏。保存基本完好，印面有污迹。

中华医学会 / 上海中医药大学医史博物馆藏

The square seal was a personal seal. Being quadrate and with the red seal characters in smooth and flowing style, the seal is exquisitely carved. The knob is in the shape of a vivid design with two lions playing with a ball. The seal was collected in 1962 and is still in good condition except for some stains on the surface. Preserved in Chinese Medical Association/ Museum of Chinese Medicine, Shanghai University of Traditional Chinese Medicine

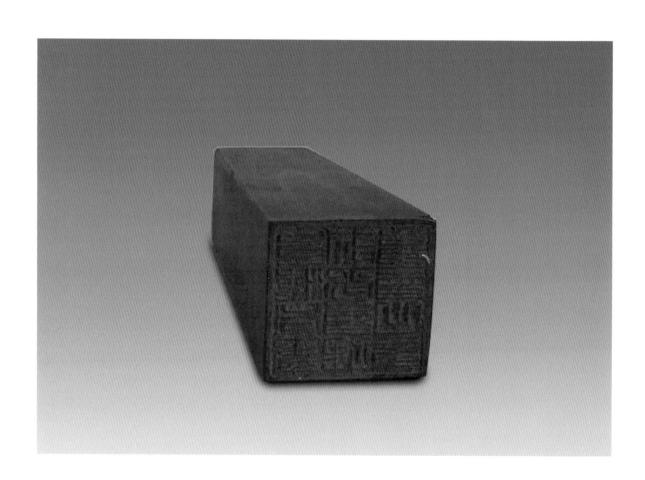

上海市医师公会理事会章

近现代

牛角质

印面边长 2.1 厘米，高 5.6 厘米

Official Seal of Trustee Council of Shanghai Physician Union

Modern Times

Ox Horn

Side Length 2.1 cm/ Height 5.6 cm

方形，为公章。该藏为公会所属理事会章。

1955 年入藏，基本完好，印面有污迹。

中华医学会 / 上海中医药大学医史博物馆藏

The quadrate official seal was utilized by Trustee Council of Shanghai Physicians Union. It was collected in 1955 and is still in good condition except for some stains on the surface. Preserved in Chinese Medical Association/ Museum of Chinese Medicine, Shanghai University of Traditional Chinese Medicine

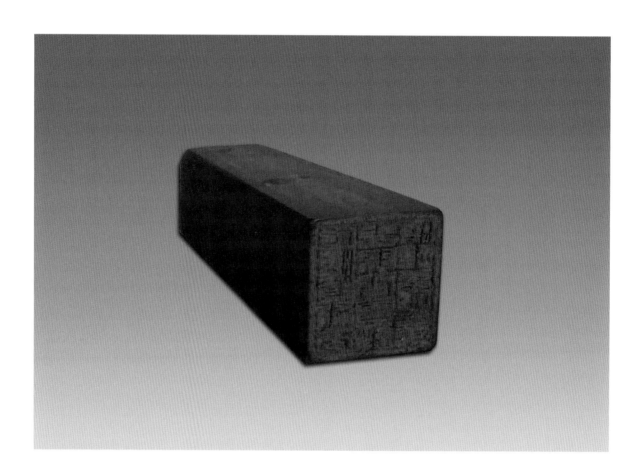

上海特别市医师公会经济理事牛角方章

近现代

牛角质

边长 1.9 厘米，宽（厚）1.9 厘米，高 5.4 厘米

Quadrate Horn Seal of Economic Council of Shanghai Special City Physicians' Union

Modern Times

Ox Horn

Side Length 1.9 cm/ Thickness 1.9 cm/ Height 5.4 cm

印面正方形，为公章。印面朱文刻"上海特别市医师公会经济理事之章"，留边框。1955 年入藏，保存清洁完好。

中华医学会／上海中医药大学医史博物馆藏

The official seal surface is square and has a rim. It is inscribed with red Chinese characters "Seal of Economic Council of Shanghai Special City Physicians' Union". The seal was collected in 1955 and is still in good condition.

Preserved in Chinese Medical Association/ Museum of Chinese Medicine, Shanghai University of Traditional Chinese Medicine

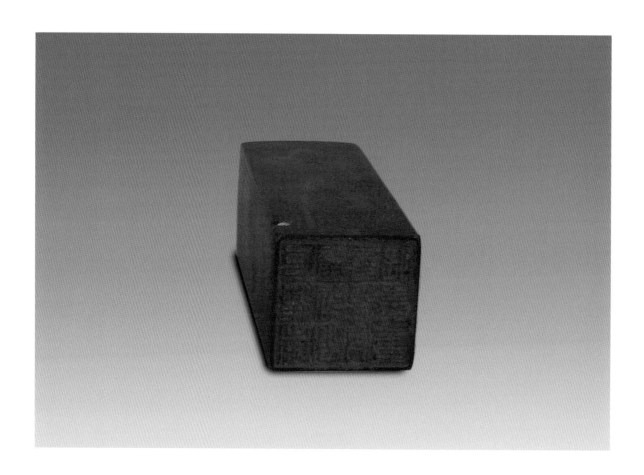

上海市医师公会经济理事章

近现代

牛角质

边长 2.2 厘米，高 6.95 厘米

Seal of Economic Council of Shanghai Physicians' Union

Modern Times

Ox Horn

Side Length 2.2 cm/ Height 6.95 cm

方形，为公章。该藏为医师公会经济理事章。

1955 年入藏，保存基本完好，印面有污迹。

中华医学会 / 上海中医药大学医史博物馆藏

The quadrate official seal was utilized by the Economic Council of Shanghai Physicians' Union. It was collected in 1955 and is still in good condition except for some stains on the surface.

Preserved in Chinese Medical Association/ Museum of Chinese Medicine, Shanghai University of Traditional Chinese Medicine

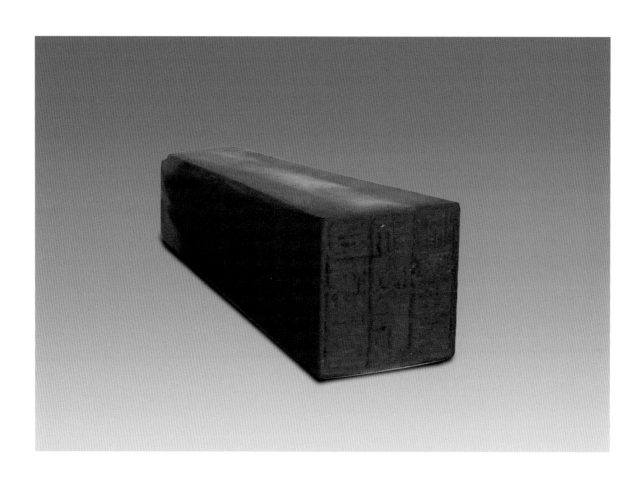

上海市医师公会经济委员章

近现代

牛角质

边长 2.05 厘米，高 5.7 厘米

Seal of Economic Council of Shanghai Physicians' Union

Modern Times

Ox Horn

Side Length 2.05 cm/ Height 5.7 cm

方形，为公章。该藏为公会所属经济委员章。

1955 年入藏，保存基本完好，印面有污迹。

中华医学会 / 上海中医药大学医史博物馆藏

The quadrate official seal was utilized by the
Economic Council of Shanghai Physicians'
Union. It was collected in 1955 and is still in
good condition except for some stains on the
surface.

Preserved in Chinese Medical Association/
Museum of Chinese Medicine, Shanghai
University of Traditional Chinese Medicine

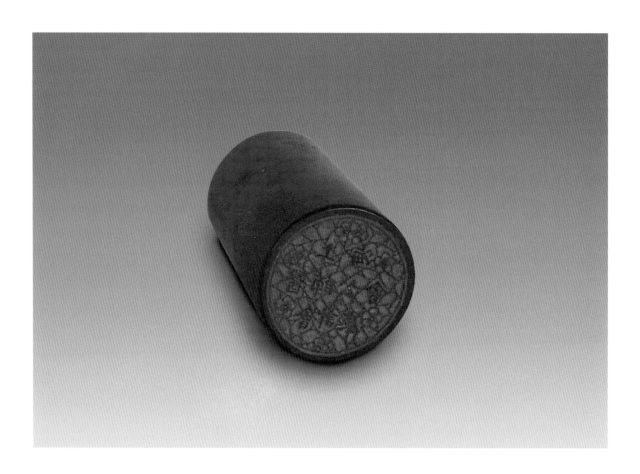

上海医师公会会计处牛角圆章

近现代

牛角质

直径 3 厘米，高 5.2 厘米

Ox-horn Circular Seal for Accounting Department of Shanghai Physicians' Union

Modern Times

Ox Horn

Diameter 3 cm/ Height 5.2 cm

印面圆形，为公章。印章刻"上海医师公会会计处"，分三行，无界格线，但整个印面刻梅花网格纹。1955 年入藏，保存完好。

中华医学会 / 上海中医药大学医史博物馆藏

The circular surface official seal was for official purpose and is incised with "Accounting Department of Shanghai Physicians' Union" in three rows without boundary line. But the whole surface is carved with the design of plum flowers. The seal was collected in 1955 and is still in good condition.

Preserved in Chinese Medical Association/ Museum of Chinese Medicine, Shanghai University of Traditional Chinese Medicine

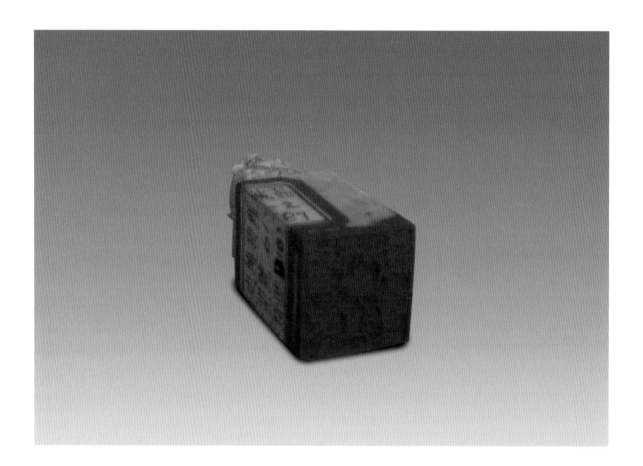

医史研究组藏书章

近现代

象牙质

边长 2.1 厘米，高 4.91 厘米

Seal of Library of Medicine History Research Group

Modern Times

Ivory

Side Length 2.1 cm/ Height 4.91 cm

方形，为公章。该章为朱孔阳先生刻制。印钮为兽钮。医史研究
组是中华医学会所属的一个研究小组。朱孔阳（1892－1986），
字云裳，上海松江人。早年习医，雅好收藏金石书画，善鉴别文物。
1953 年，应聘于中华医学会上海分会医史博物馆。1972 年，任
上海文史馆馆员，著有《殷墟文字考释校正》等书。1961 年入藏，
保存基本完好，印面有污迹。

中华医学会 / 上海中医药大学医史博物馆藏

The quadrate official seal was engraved by Mr. Zhu Kongyang. The
knob is in the shape of an animal. The Medicine History Research
Group was one of the research institutes of Chinese Medical
Association. Mr. Zhu Kongyang (1892-1986), styled his name as
Yunshang, was born in Songjiang, Shanghai. He studied medicine
in his early years and one of his favorite hobbies was the collection
of ancient metals, stones, calligraphy and paintings. He was good at
identifying antiques. In 1953, he was employed by the Museum of
Medicine History, Shanghai Branch of Chinese Medical Association.
In 1972, he became a librarian of Shanghai Research Institute of
Culture and History. He had written the books such as *Textual
Research, Explanation, and Correction of Characters in Yin Ruins* of
the Shang Dynasty and so on. The seal was collected in 1961 and is
still in good condition except for some stains on the surface.
Preserved in Chinese Medical Association/ Museum of Chinese
Medicine, Shanghai University of Traditional Chinese Medicine

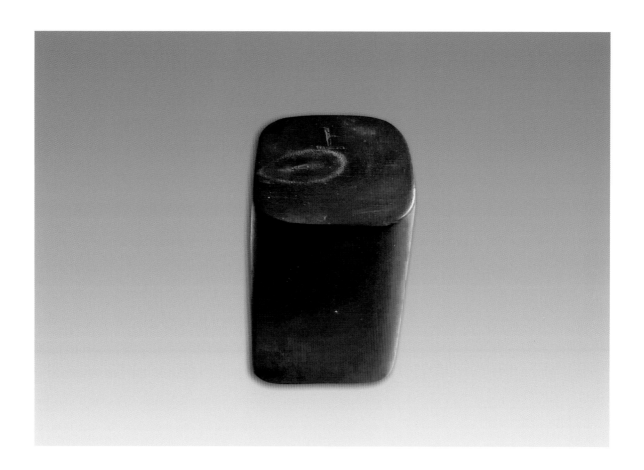

永和药号印章

近现代

木质

边长 3.6 厘米，高 5.6 厘米

Stamp of Yonghe Pharmacy

Modern times

Wood

Side Length 3.6 cm/ Height 5.6 cm

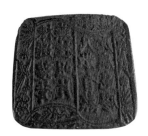

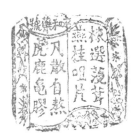

红木质，印章上刻有"永和药号""精选参茸燕桂咀片""丸散自熬虎鹿龟胶"。1948年虞子明、聂友僧、皮清心、叶森林在株洲开设永和药号。

新昌县天姥中医博物馆藏

The stamp is made of red wood, engraved with inscriptions of (Yong He Yao Hao), (Jing Xuan Shen Rong Yan Gui Ju Pian) and (Wan San Zi Ao Hu Lu Gui Jiao) which indicate the names of the Pharmacy and medicines. In 1948, Yu Ziming, Nie Youseng, Pi Qingxin and Ye Senlin set up Yonghe Pharmacy in Zhuzhou.
Preserved in Tianmu Traditional Chinese Medicine Museum of Xinchang County

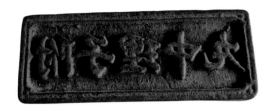

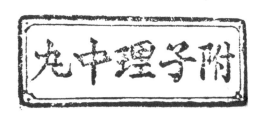

附子理中丸印章

近现代

木质

长 5.5 厘米，宽 2 厘米，高 4 厘米

阳文，刻"附子理中丸"，绍兴老药铺征集。

新昌县天姥中医博物馆藏

Stamp of FuziLizhong Pill

Modern times

Wood

Length 5.5 cm/ Width 2 cm/ Height 4 cm

The characters cut in relief are reading "Fu Zi Li Zhong Wan" which means the functions of the pill and it was collected from old medicine shop in Shaoxing.

Preserved in Tianmu Traditional Chinese Medicine Museum of Xinchang County

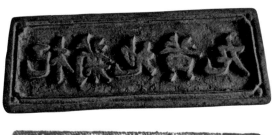

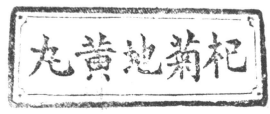

杞菊地黄丸印章

近现代

木质

长 5.5 厘米，宽 2 厘米，高 4 厘米

阳文，刻"杞菊地黄丸"，绍兴老药铺征集。

新昌县天姥中医博物馆藏

Stamp of QijuDihuang Pill

Modern times

Wood

Length 5.5 cm/ Width 2 cm/ Height 4 cm

Characters cut in relief are reading "Qi ju Di huang Wan" which means the functions of the pill and it was collected from old medicine shop in Shaoxing.

Preserved in Tianmu Traditional Chinese Medicine Museum of Xinchang County

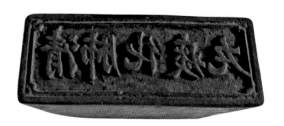

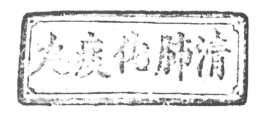

清肺化痰丸印章

近现代

木质

长 5.5 厘米，宽 2 厘米，高 4 厘米

Stamp of Qingfeihuatan Pill

Modern times

Wood

Length 5.5 cm/ Width 2 cm/ Height 4 cm

阳文，刻"清肺化痰丸"，绍兴老药铺征集。

新昌县天姥中医博物馆藏

Characters cut in relief are reading "Qing Fei Hua Tan Wan" which means the functions of the pill and it was collected from old medicine shop in Shaoxing.

Preserved in Tianmu Traditional Chinese Medicine Museum of Xinchang County

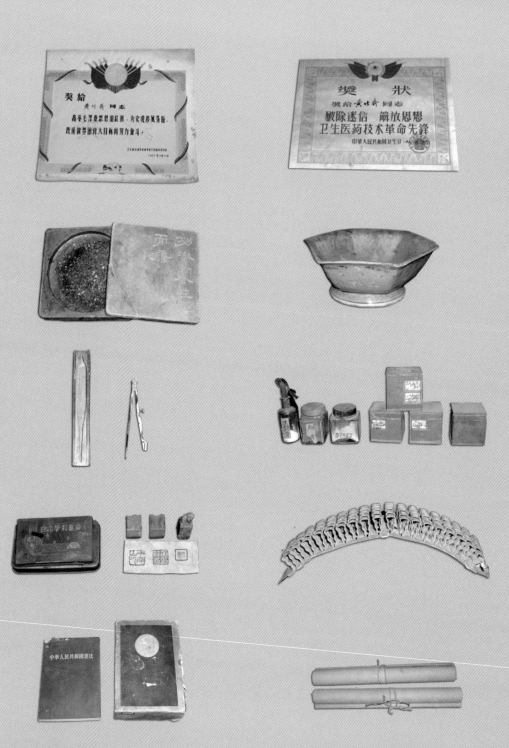

黄竹斋遗物

近现代

重 7500 克

砚台1方，印章3枚，六棱碗1个，健脑器1个，药瓶7个，圆规1个，《毛泽东选集》3本，《中华人名共和国宪法》1本，印盒1个，字画2副，奖状2张。医疗用具。陕西省西安市黄竹斋家人捐赠。

陕西医史博物馆藏

Huang Zhuzhai's Mementos

Modern Times

Weight 7500 g

All the mementos include a inkslab, three seals, a hexagonal bowl, a brain fitness device, seven medicine bottles, a dividers, three books entitled Chairmen Mao's excerption, a Constitution of the People's Republic of China, 2 seal boxes, 2 scrolls of paintings, and 2 certificates of merit. Some are for medical purpose. These were donated by Huang Zhuzhai's family in Xi'an City, Shaanxi Province.

Preserved in Shaanxi Museum of Medicine History

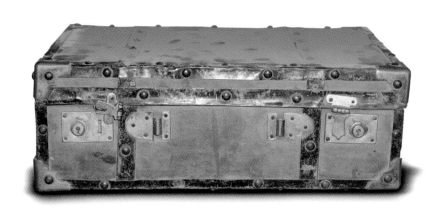

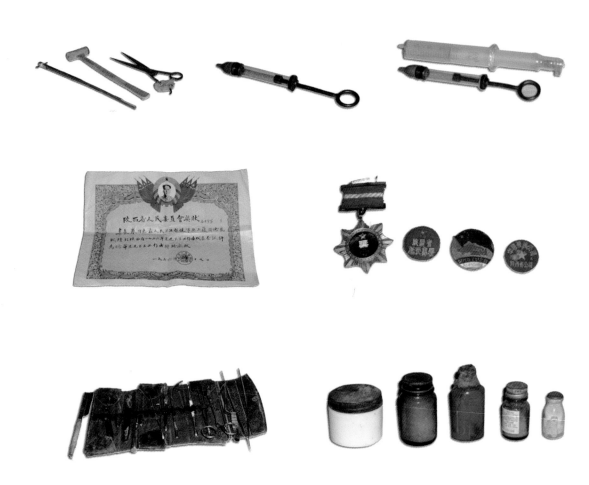

李长春药箱

近现代

木质、铁质

长 39 厘米，宽 23.5 厘米，高 13 厘米，重 3900 克

药箱为长方形，内层贴棉布，外包有铁皮，四个外角有铜角饰。内装药标签 9 张，李长春获 1956 年陕西省人民政府奖状 1 张，奖章 4 枚，医疗器械 28 件，用药处方 28 张，药物 31 种，绑腿一副 2 件，均为李长春在延安保健药社使用过的器物。出诊箱、药箱稍残，其余基本完整。

陕西医史博物馆藏

Li Changchun's Medicine Case

Modern Times

Wood and Iron

Length 39 cm/Width 23.5 cm/Height 13 cm/Weight 3,900 g

The case is rectangular. The inner layer is pasted with cotton, and the exterior is wrapped with iron sheet. The four edges of the case are decorated with copper ornaments. Inside the case, there are 9 medicine labels, a certificate to honor Mr. Li Changchun by the Shaanxi People's Government in 1956, 4 medals, 28 medical apparatus and instruments, 28 prescriptions, 31 kinds of medicine and a pair of leggings, which were used by Mr. Li Changchun when he was working in Yan'an Health-protection Agency. The home visit medicine box and the medicine chest are slightly damaged, but the others are still in good condition.

Preserved in Shaanxi Museum of Medicine History

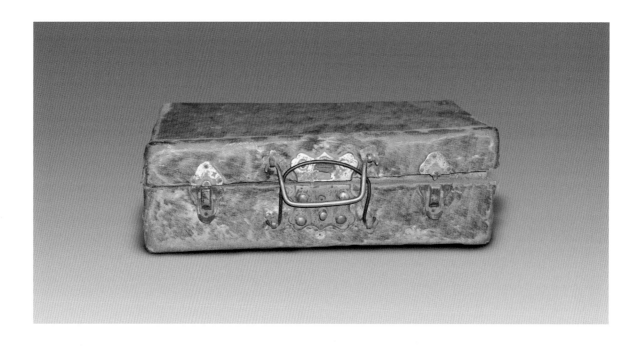

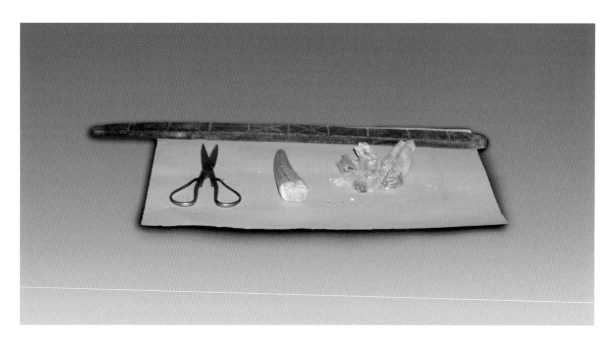

牛皮药箱

近现代

木质、皮质

长 35 厘米，宽 20 厘米，高 12 厘米，重 1500 克

木质药箱，外全包牛皮，内有木尺 1 件，剪刀 1 件，药物 2 种。用于出诊时盛装药物。陕北征集。基本完整。

陕西医史博物馆藏

Cattlehide Medicine Case

Modern Times

Wood and Leather

Length 35 cm/ Width 20 cm/ Height 12 cm/ Weight 1,500 g

The wooden case is entirely wrapped with the cattle hides. In the case, there is a wooden ruler, a pair of scissors and two kinds of medicines. The case was for carrying medicines when going out for a home visit. It was collected in Northern Shaanxi Province and is still in good condition.

Preserved in Shaanxi Museum of Medicine History

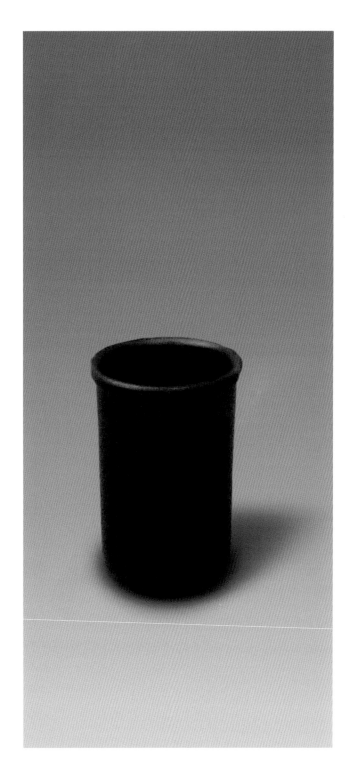

火罐

近现代

角质

直径 4.8 厘米，高 7.1 厘米

Cupping Jar

Modern Times

Horn

Diameter 4.8 cm/ Height 7.1 cm

直杯形。该藏是中医用火来灸治疾病的用具，称火罐。医用。1958 年入藏，保存基本完好。

中华医学会／上海中医药大学医史博物馆藏

The cupping jar is shaped as a straight cup. The collection was utilized for treating diseases by moxibustion in Traditional Chinese Medicine. It was collected in 1958 and is still in good condition.

Preserved in Chinese Medical Association/ Museum of Chinese Medicine, Shanghai University of Traditional Chinese Medicine

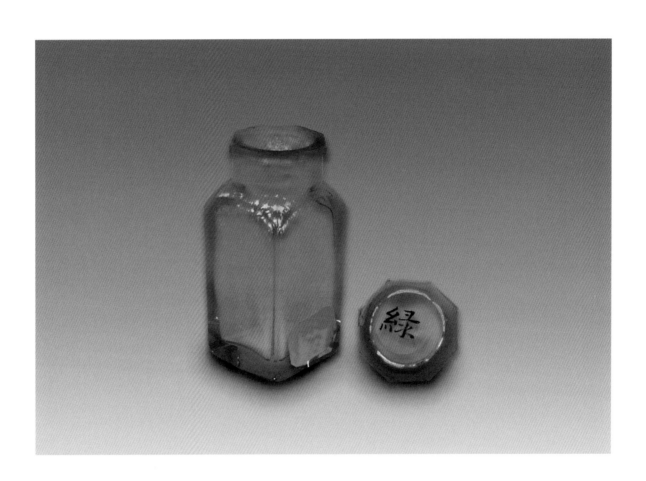

玻璃药瓶

近现代

玻璃质

边长 3 厘米，通高 7.3 厘米

Glass Medicine Bottle

Modern Times

Glass

Side Length 3 cm/ Height 7.3 cm

方瓶形。该组药瓶为南翔张志方中药室红木药箱内配玻璃药瓶之一，平底磨砂口，上配磨砂八角玻璃瓶盖，每个瓶盖上粘有药名标签，质地做工均佳，造型美观。盛药器具。1959 年入藏，保存基本完好。

中华医学会 / 上海中医药大学医史博物馆藏

The bottle is square-shaped. The collection is one of the glass medicine bottles equipped in the mahogany medicine chest in Zhang Zhifang Traditional Chinese Medicine Store at Nanxiang. The bottle has a flat bottom and a frosting mouth and a frosting octagonal glass lid. A label of the medicine name is pasted on the lid. With beautiful designs, the bottle is of good quality and fine workmanship. It was utilized for storing medicines. It was collected in 1959 and is still in good condition.
Preserved in Chinese Medical Association/ Museum of Chinese Medicine, Shanghai University of Traditional Chinese Medicine

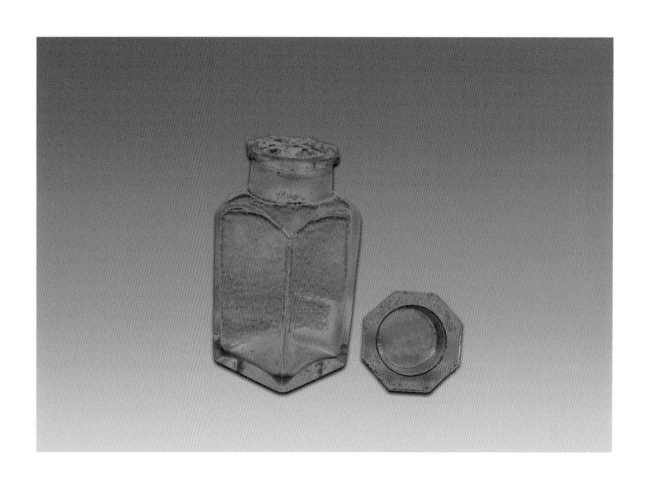

玻璃药瓶

近现代

玻璃质

边长 3 厘米，通高 7.3 厘米

Glass Medicine Bottle

Modern Times

Glass

Side Length 3 cm/ Height 7.3 cm

方瓶形。该组药瓶为南翔张志方中药室红木
药箱内配玻璃药瓶之一，平底磨砂口，上配
磨砂八角玻璃瓶盖，每个瓶盖上粘有药名标
签，质地做工均佳，造型美观。盛药器具。
1959 年入藏，保存基本完好。

中华医学会 / 上海中医药大学医史博物馆藏

The bottle is square-shaped. The collection
is one of the glass medicine bottles equipped
in the mahogany medicine chest in Zhang
Zhifang Traditional Chinese Medicine Store at
Nanxiang. The bottle has a flat bottom and a
frosting mouth and a frosting octagonal glass
lid. A label of the medicine name is pasted on
the lid. With beautiful designs, the bottle is
of good quality and fine workmanship. It was
utilized for storing medicines. It was collected
in 1959 and is still in good condition.
Preserved in Chinese Medical Association/
Museum of Chinese Medicine, Shanghai
University of Traditional Chinese Medicine

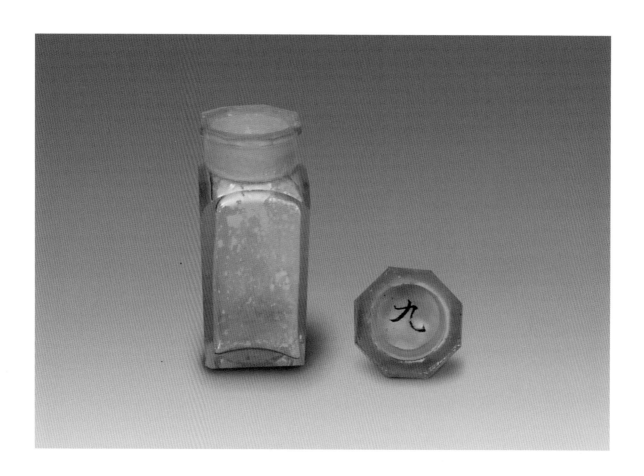

玻璃药瓶

近现代

玻璃质

边长 3 厘米，通高 7.3 厘米

Glass Medicine Bottle

Modern Times

Glass

Side Length 3 cm/ Height 7.3 cm

方瓶形。该组药瓶为南翔张志方中药室红木药
箱内配玻璃药瓶之一，平底磨砂口，上配磨砂
八角玻瓶盖，每个瓶盖上粘有药名标签，质地
做工均佳，造型美观。盛药器具。1959年入藏，
保存基本完好。

中华医学会 / 上海中医药大学医史博物馆藏

The bottle is square-shaped. The collection
is one of the glass medicine bottles equipped
in the mahogany medicine chest in Zhang
Zhifang Traditional Chinese Medicine Store at
Nanxiang. The bottle has a flat bottom and a
frosting mouth and a frosting octagonal glass
lid. A label of the medicine name is pasted on
the lid. With beautiful designs, the bottle is
of good quality and fine workmanship. It was
utilized for storing medicines. It was collected
in 1959 and is still in good condition.
Preserved in Chinese Medical Association/
Museum of Chinese Medicine, Shanghai
University of Traditional Chinese Medicine

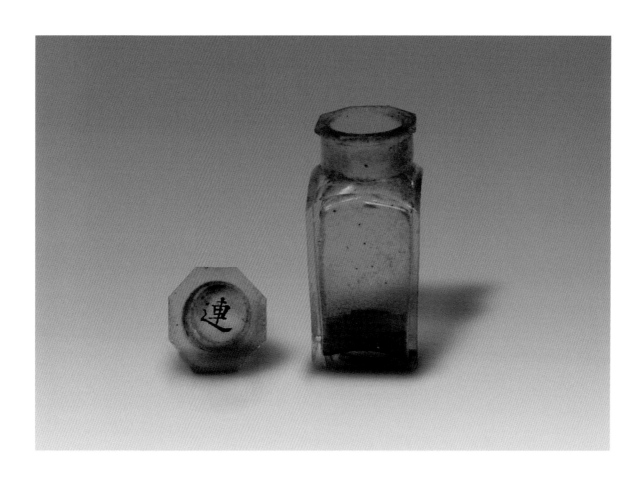

玻璃药瓶

近现代

玻璃质

边长 3 厘米，通高 7.3 厘米

Glass Medicine Bottle

Modern Times

Glass

Side Length 3 cm/ Height 7.3 cm

方瓶形。该组药瓶为南翔张志方中药室红木
药箱内配玻璃药瓶之一，平底磨砂口，上配
磨砂八角玻璃瓶盖，每个瓶盖上粘有药名标
签，质地做工均佳，造型美观。盛药器具。
1959 年入藏，保存基本完好。

中华医学会 / 上海中医药大学医史博物馆藏

The bottle is square-shaped. The collection
is one of the glass medicine bottles equipped
in the mahogany medicine chest in Zhang
Zhifang Traditional Chinese Medicine Store at
Nanxiang. The bottle has a flat bottom and a
frosting mouth and a frosting octagonal glass
lid. A label of the medicine name is pasted on
the lid. With beautiful designs, the bottle is
of good quality and fine workmanship. It was
utilized for storing medicines. It was collected
in 1959 and is still in good condition.
Preserved in Chinese Medical Association/
Museum of Chinese Medicine, Shanghai
University of Traditional Chinese Medicine

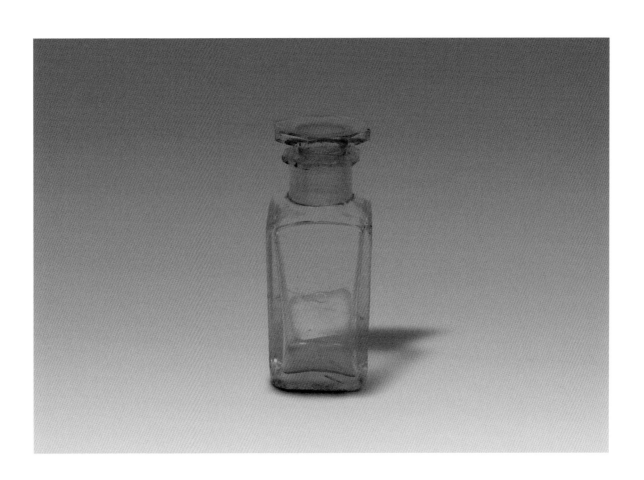

玻璃药瓶

近现代

玻璃质

边长 3 厘米，通高 7.3 厘米

Glass Medicine Bottle

Modern Times

Glass

Side Length 3 cm/ Height 7.3 cm

方瓶形。该组药瓶为南翔张志方中药室红木
药箱内配玻璃药瓶之一，平底磨砂口，上配
磨砂八角玻璃瓶盖，每个瓶盖上粘有药名标
签，质地做工均佳，造型美观。盛药器具。
1959 年入藏，保存基本完好。

中华医学会 / 上海中医药大学医史博物馆藏

The bottle is square-shaped. The collection
is one of the glass medicine bottles equipped
in the mahogany medicine chest in Zhang
Zhifang Traditional Chinese Medicine Store at
Nanxiang. The bottle has a flat bottom and a
frosting mouth and a frosting octagonal glass
lid. A label of the medicine name is pasted on
the lid. With beautiful designs, the bottle is
of good quality and fine workmanship. It was
utilized for storing medicines. It was collected
in 1959 and is still in good condition.
Preserved in Chinese Medical Association/
Museum of Chinese Medicine, Shanghai
University of Traditional Chinese Medicine

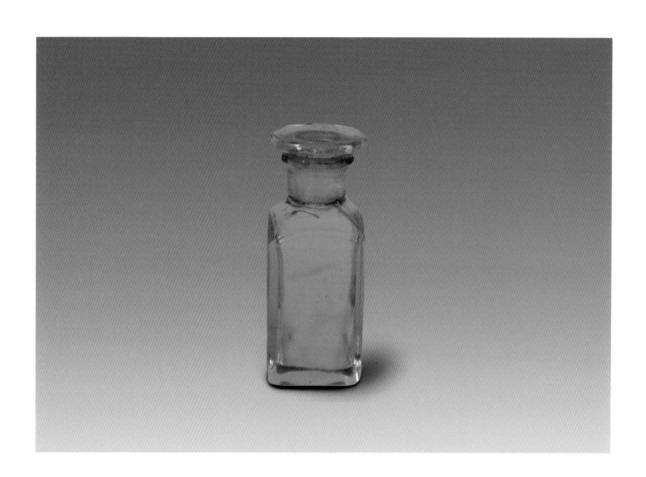

玻璃药瓶

近现代

玻璃质

边长 3 厘米，通高 7.3 厘米

Glass Medicine Bottle

Modern Times

Glass

Side Length 3 cm/ Height 7.3 cm

方瓶形。该组药瓶为南翔张志方中药室红木
药箱内配玻璃药瓶之一，平底磨砂口，上配
磨砂八角玻璃瓶盖，每个瓶盖上粘有药名标
签，质地做工均佳，造型美观。盛药器具。
1959 年入藏，保存基本完好。

中华医学会 / 上海中医药大学医史博物馆藏

The bottle is square-shaped. The collection
is one of the glass medicine bottles equipped
in the mahogany medicine chest in Zhang
Zhifang Traditional Chinese Medicine Store
at Nanxiang. The bottle has a flat bottom, a
frosting mouth and a frosting octagonal glass
lid. A label of the medicine name is pasted on
the lid. With beautiful designs, the bottle is
of good quality and fine workmanship. It was
utilized for storing medicines. It was collected
in 1959 and is still in good condition.
Preserved in Chinese Medical Association/
Museum of Chinese Medicine, Shanghai
University of Traditional Chinese Medicine

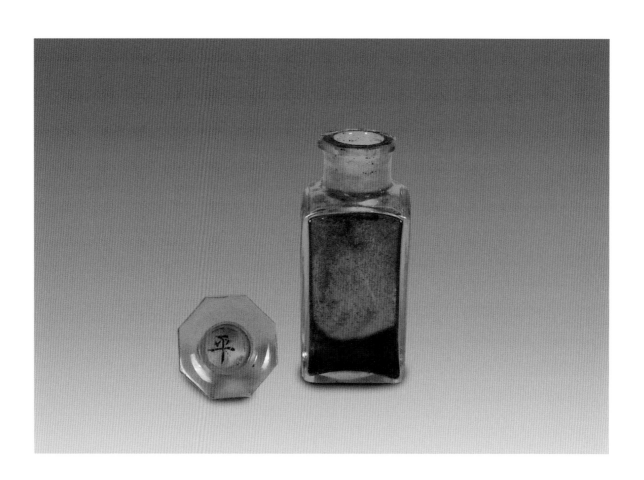

玻璃药瓶

近现代

玻璃质

边长 3 厘米，通高 7.3 厘米

Glass Medicine Bottle

Modern Times

Glass

Side Length 3 cm/ Height 7.3 cm

方瓶形。该组药瓶为南翔张志方中药室红木
药箱内配玻璃药瓶之一，平底磨砂口，上配
磨砂八角玻璃瓶盖，每个瓶盖上粘有药名标
签，质地做工均佳，造型美观。盛药器具。
1959 年入藏，保存基本完好。

中华医学会 / 上海中医药大学医史博物馆藏

The bottle is square-shaped. The collection
is one of the glass medicine bottles equipped
in the mahogany medicine chest in Zhang
Zhifang Traditional Chinese Medicine Store
at Nanxiang. The bottle has a flat bottom, a
frosting mouth and a frosting octagonal glass
lid. A label of the medicine name is pasted on
the lid. With beautiful designs, the bottle is
of good quality and fine workmanship. It was
utilized for storing medicines. It was collected
in 1959 and is still in good condition.
Preserved in Chinese Medical Association/
Museum of Chinese Medicine, Shanghai
University of Traditional Chinese Medicine

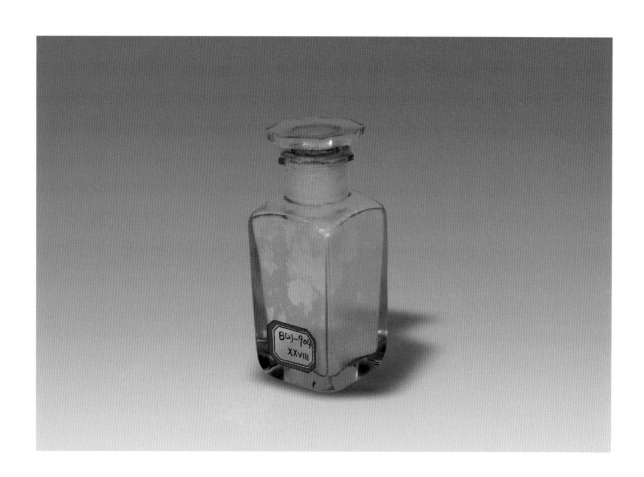

玻璃药瓶

近现代

玻璃质

边长 3 厘米，通高 7.3 厘米

Glass Medicine Bottle

Modern Times

Glass

Side Length 3 cm/ Height 7.3 cm

方瓶形。该组药瓶为南翔张志方中药室红木药箱内配玻璃药瓶之一，平底磨砂口，上配磨砂八角玻璃瓶盖，每个瓶盖上粘有药名标签，质地做工均佳，造型美观。盛药器具。1959 年入藏，保存基本完好。

中华医学会 / 上海中医药大学医史博物馆藏

The bottle is square-shaped. The collection is one of the glass medicine bottles equipped in the mahogany medicine chest in Zhang Zhifang Traditional Chinese Medicine Store at Nanxiang. The bottle has a flat bottom, a frosting mouth and a frosting octagonal glass lid. A label of the medicine name is pasted on the lid. With beautiful designs, the bottle is of good quality and fine workmanship. It was utilized for storing medicines. It was collected in 1959 and is still in good condition.
Preserved in Chinese Medical Association/ Museum of Chinese Medicine, Shanghai University of Traditional Chinese Medicine

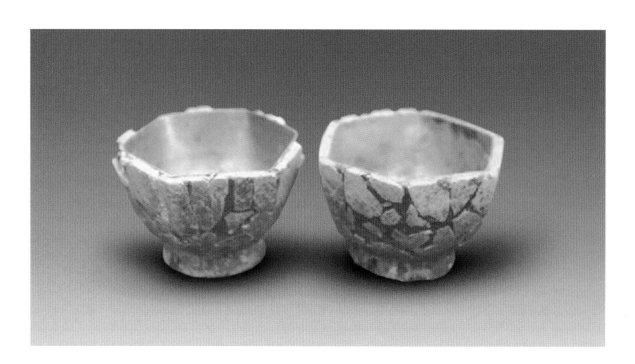

雄精锡胎六角酒杯

近现代

石质包锡

左：通高 3.5 厘米，外口径 5.1 厘米，底口径 2.9 厘米，边长 2.8 厘米，重 56 克

右：通高 3.6 厘米，外口径 5.5 厘米，底口径 3.1 厘米，边长 2.95 厘米，重 66 克

Hexagonal Realgar Wine Cups with Tin Base

Modern Times

Stone covered with Tin

The Left One: Height 3.5 cm/ Mouth Outer Diameter 5.1 cm/ Mouth Bottom Diameter 2.9 cm/Side length 2.8 cm/ Weight 56 g

The Right One: Height 3.6 cm/ Mouth Outer Diameter 5.5 cm/ Mouth Bottom Diameter 3.1 cm/Side length 2.95 cm/ Weight 66 g

雄精即雄黄一种中药，雄黄制锡胎六角酒杯，六
角形，圈足，一种用中药材雕刻的艺术品。

广东中医药博物馆藏

Realgar is a kind of traditional Chinese herbal
medicine. This wine cup with a ring foot is
hexagonal. It is an artwork carved with traditional
Chinese herbal medicine.

Preserved in Guangzhou Chinese Medicine Museum

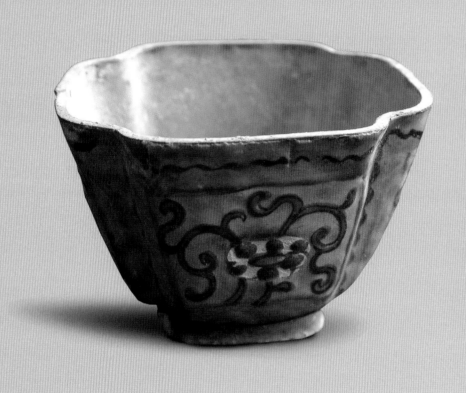

酒杯

近现代

石质包锡

口径 4.5 厘米，高 3 厘米

方形景泰蓝酒杯。

江苏省中医药博物馆藏

Wine Cup

Modern Times

Stone covered with Tin

Mouth Diameter 4.5 cm/ Height 3 cm

It is a square cloisonn wine cup.

Preserved in Jiangsu Museum of Traditional

Chinese Medicine

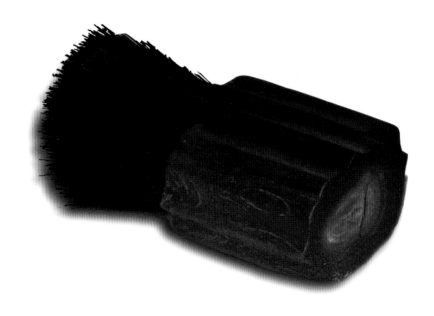

药帚

近现代

角质、鬃毛

长 9.8 厘米，宽 4.95 厘米

帚状。医用。帚柄为椭圆柱形角制，帚刷毛为黑色鬃毛。1956 年入藏。保存基本完好。

中华医学会 / 上海中医药大学医史博物馆藏

Medicine Brush

Modern Times

Horn and Horsehair

Length 9.8 cm/ Width 4.95 cm

The brush is in the shape of a broom for medical use. The handle of the brush is made of elliptical pillar-shaped horn, and the brush hair is black horsehair. The brush was collected in 1956 and is kept in good condition.

Preserved in Chinese Medical Association/ Museum of Chinese Medicine, Shanghai University of Traditional Chinese Medicine

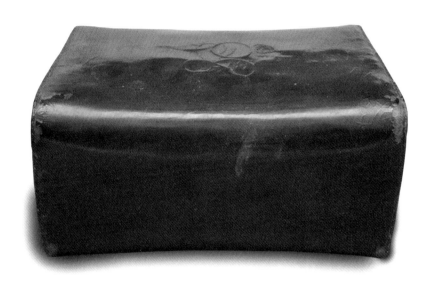

脉枕

近现代

皮质

长 11 厘米，宽 7 厘米，高 7.5 厘米

皮上髹层红漆。由民间征集。

成都中医药大学中医药传统文化博物馆藏

Wrist Cushion for Pulse-taking

Modern Times

Leather

Length 11 cm/ Width 7 cm/ Height 7.5 cm

The leather wrist cushion is lacquered with red paint. It was collected from a private owner.

Preserved in Museum of Traditional Chinese Medicine Culture, Chengdu University of Traditional Chinese Medicine

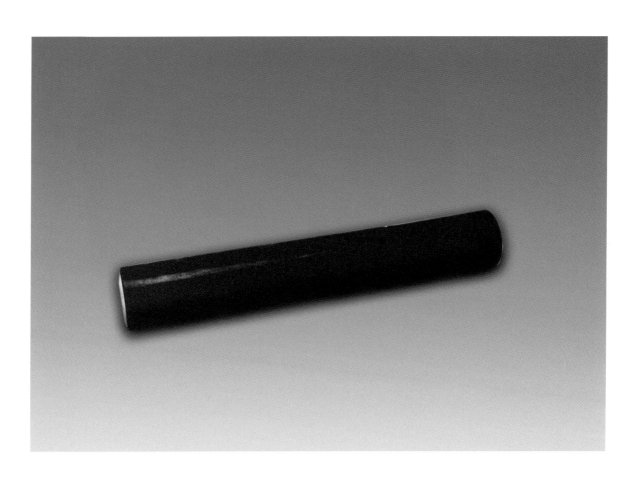

针筒

近现代

骨质

直径 2.5 厘米，长 13.5 厘米

Needle Container

Modern Times

Bone

Diameter 2.5 cm/ Length 13.5 cm

黑褐色，器物外表呈现骨质纹理。造型简捷
实用，是医生用来装置针灸用针的工具。由
民间征集。

　　成都中医药大学中医药传统文化博物馆藏

The container is black brown. The surface of
the item takes the form of bone texture patterns.
Simple but practical, it was utilized for storing
acupuncture needles and was collected from a
private owner.

Preserved in Museum of Traditional Chinese
Medicine Culture, Chengdu University of
Traditional Chinese Medicine

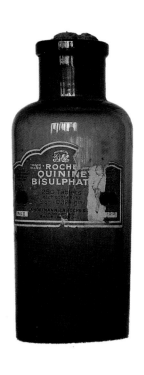
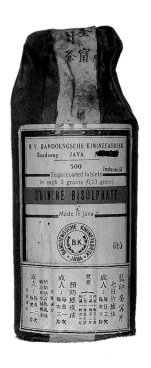

印尼奎宁药瓶

近现代

玻璃质

高 15 厘米

印度尼西亚的奎宁，尚未开封。

上海医药文献博物馆民国馆藏

Bottle of Indonesia Quinine

Modern Times

Glass

Height 15 cm

Quinine from Indonesia, unopened

Preserved in the Museum of Republic of China/Shanghai Medical Literature Museum

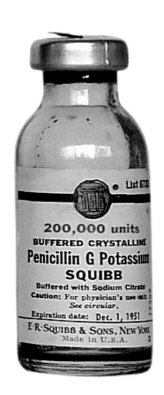

施贵宝盘尼西林药瓶

近现代

玻璃质

高 5 厘米

施贵宝盘尼西林，1948 年出品。

上海医药文献博物馆民国馆藏

Medicine Bottle of Penicillin of Bristol-Myers Squibb

Modern Times

Glass

Height 5 cm

Penicillin of Bristol-Myers Squibb, produced in 1948.

Preserved in the Museum of Republic of China/Shanghai Medical Literature Museum

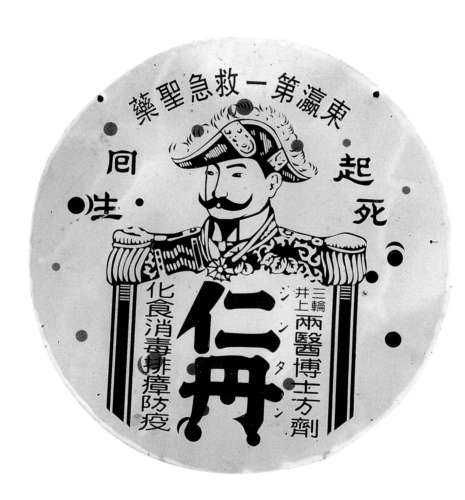

仁丹广告

近现代

搪瓷质

直径 50 厘米

"翘胡子仁丹"搪瓷广告牌，全球最大，直径 50 厘米。20 世纪 20 年代末，日本蓄意向中国发动侵略战争，千方百计地刺探和搜集中国的情报。广告牌中胡子尖所指的方向，就是需要刺探中国的机密所在。日本侵略者根据"翘胡子仁丹"暗示的位置，向中国的目标发起攻击。

上海医药文献博物馆民国馆藏

Advertisements of Jintan

Modern Times

Enamel

Diameter 50 cm

It's a 50cm-long enamel advertisement board of "Tilted Beard" brand Jintan, the largest in the world. In late 1920s, Japan deliberately launched an invasion to China, painstakingly spying and collecting intelligence. The direction of the tip of the tilted beard points to where the intelligence lay. The Japanese invaders would then attack the targets based on the direction of the beard's tip.

Preserved in the Museum of Republic of China/Shanghai Medical Literature Museum

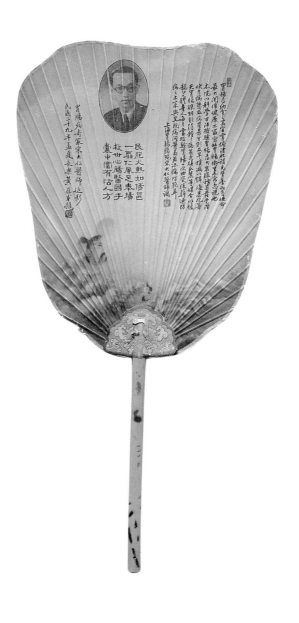

宋大仁广告扇

近现代

塑料质

长 35 厘米，宽 20 厘米

1940 年，上海胃肠病院宋大仁医师为自己和医院制作的广告扇。广州中医药博物馆能有今日之成就，最要感谢的便是宋教授。

上海医药文献博物馆民国馆藏

Advertising Fan of Song Daren

Modern Times

Plastic

Length 35 cm/ Width 20 cm

In 1940, Dr. Song Daren in Shanghai Gastroenteropathy Hospital made an advertising fan for himself and the hospital. It was Professor Song to whom the Guangzhou Traditional Chinese Medicine Museum's success owes.

Preserved in the Museum of Republic of China/Shanghai Medical Literature Museum

索 引

（馆藏地按拼音字母排序）

中山陵园管理局

Index

Sun Yatsen Mausoleum Park

参考文献

[1] 李经纬 . 中国古代医史图录 [M]. 北京：人民卫生出版社，1992.

[2] 傅维康，李经纬，林昭庚 . 中国医学通史：文物图谱卷 [M]. 北京：人民卫生出版社，2000.

[3] 和中浚，吴鸿洲 . 中华医学文物图集 [M]. 成都：四川人民出版社，2001.

[4] 上海中医药博物馆 . 上海中医药博物馆馆藏珍品 [M]. 上海：上海科学技术出版社，2013.

[5] 西藏自治区博物馆 . 西藏博物馆 [M]. 北京：五洲传播出版社，2005.

[6] 崔乐泉 . 中国古代体育文物图录：中英文本 [M]. 北京：中华书局，2000.

[7] 张金明，陆雪春 . 中国古铜镜鉴赏图录 [M]. 北京：中国民族摄影艺术出版社，2002.

[8] 文物精华编辑委员会 . 文物精华 [M]. 北京：文物出版社，1964.

[9] 谭维四 . 湖北出土文物精华 [M]. 武汉：湖北教育出版社，2001.

[10] 常州市博物馆 . 常州文物精华 [M]. 北京：文物出版社，1998.

[11] 镇江博物馆 . 镇江文物精华 [M]. 合肥：黄山书社，1997.

[12] 贵州省文化厅，贵州省博物馆 . 贵州文物精华 [M]. 贵阳：贵州人民出版社，2005.

[13] 徐良玉 . 扬州馆藏文物精华 [M]. 南京：江苏古籍出版社，2001.

[14] 昭陵博物馆，陕西历史博物馆 . 昭陵文物精华 [M]. 西安：陕西人民美术出版社，1991.

[15] 南通博物苑 . 南通博物苑文物精华 [M]. 北京：文物出版社，2005.

[16] 邯郸市文物研究所 . 邯郸文物精华 [M]. 北京：文物出版社，2005.

[17] 张秀生，刘友恒，聂连顺，等 . 中国河北正定文物精华 [M]. 北京：文化艺术出版社，1998.

[18] 陕西省咸阳市文物局 . 咸阳文物精华 [M]. 北京：文物出版社，2002.

[19] 安阳市文物管理局 . 安阳文物精华 [M]. 北京：文物出版社，2004.

[20] 深圳市博物馆 . 深圳市博物馆文物精华 [M]. 北京：文物出版社，1998.

[21]《中国文物精华》编辑委员会 . 中国文物精华（1993）[M]. 北京：文物出版社，1993.

[22] 夏路，刘永生.山西省博物馆馆藏文物精华 [M].太原：山西人民出版社，1999.

[23] 文物精华编辑委员会.文物精华 [M].北京：文物出版社，1957.

[24] 山西博物院，湖北省博物馆.荆楚长歌：九连墩楚墓出土文物精华 [M].太原：山西人民出版社，2011.

[25] 刘广堂，石金鸣，宋建忠.晋国雄风：山西出土两周文物精华 [M].沈阳：万卷出版公司，2009.

[26] 沈君山，王国平，单迎红.滦平博物馆馆藏文物精华 [M].北京：中国文联出版社，2012.

[27] 张家口市博物馆.张家口市博物馆馆藏文物精华 [M].北京：科学出版社，2011.

[28] 浙江省文物考古研究所.浙江考古精华 [M].北京：文物出版社，1999.

[29] 故宫博物院.故宫雕刻珍萃 [M].北京：紫禁城出版社，2004.

[30] 故宫博物院紫禁城出版社.故宫博物院藏宝录 [M].上海：上海文艺出版社，1986.

[31] 首都博物馆.大元三都 [M].北京：科学出版社，2016.

[32] 新疆维吾尔自治区博物馆.新疆出土文物 [M].北京：文物出版社，1975.

[33] 王兴伊，段逸山.新疆出土涉医文书辑校 [M].上海：上海科学技术出版社，2016.

[34] 刘学春.刍议医药卫生文物的概念与分类标准 [J].中华中医药杂志，2016，31（11）:4406-4409.

[35] 上海古籍出版社.中国艺海 [M].上海：上海古籍出版社，1994.

[36] 紫都，岳鑫.一生必知的 200 件国宝 [M].呼和浩特：远方出版社，2005.

[37] 谭维四.湖北出土文物精华 [M].武汉：湖北教育出版社，2001.

[38] 张建青.青海彩陶收藏与鉴赏 [M].北京：中国文史出版社，2007.

[39] 银景琦.仡佬族文物 [M].南宁：广西人民出版社，2014.

[40] 廖果，梁峻，李经纬.东西方医学的反思与前瞻 [M].北京：中医古籍出版社，2002.

[41] 梁峻，张志斌，廖果，等.中华医药文明史集论 [M].北京：中医古籍出版社，2003.

[42] 郑蓉，庄乾竹，刘聪，等.中国医药文化遗产考论 [M].北京：中医古籍出版社，2005.